OBRA Nurse Aide
Skills Manual

OBRA Nurse Aide
Skills Manual

Stephanie Vaughn, R.N., M.S.N., C.R.R.N.
Mount Carmel Medical Center

Sheila A. Sorrentino, B.S.N., M.A., Ph.D.
Kankakee Community College

With 160 *illustrations*

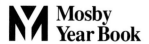
Mosby
Year Book

St. Louis   Baltimore   Boston   Chicago   London   Philadelphia   Sydney   Toronto

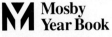

Mosby
Year Book

Dedicated to Publishing Excellence

Executive Editor Richard A. Weimer
Developmental Editor Rina A. Steinhauer
Assistant Editor Mary Beth Ryan

Printed in the United States of America.

Mosby–Year Book, Inc.
11830 Westline Industrial Drive   St. Louis, MO 63146

Library of Congress Cataloging in Publication Data
Vaughn, Stephanie, M.S.N.
　　OBRA nurse aide skills manual / Stephanie Vaughn, Sheila Sorrentin
　　　p.　cm.
　　Includes bibiliographical references and index.
　　ISBN 0-8016-6072-6
　　1. Nurses'aides--Handbooks,manuals,etc. I. Sorrentino, Sheila A.
　　II. Title.
　　　[DNLM: 1. Homes for the Aged--standards--United States-
　　-legislation. 2. Nurses' Aides—education—United States-
　　-legislation. 3. Nurses' Aides—standards—United States-
　　-legislation. 4. Nursing Homes—standards—United States-
　　-legislation. WY 33 AA1 V3ol
　　RT84.V38 1992
　　610.73—dc20
　　DNLM/DLC
　　for Library of Congress　　　　　　　　　　　　　　　　　91-25

92 93 94 95 96 CL/DC/DC 9 8 7 6 5 4 3 2 1

PREFACE

Job expectations for the nurse aide working in a nursing facility are great. Therefore, it's important that you be provided with a comprehensive text to help prepare for those requirements.

The OBRA Nurse Aide Skills Manual provides the student with current and thorough content about the OBRA requirements for the Nurse Aide Training and Competency Evaluation Program.

The contents include communication and interpersonal skills, infection control, safety and emergency procedures, and resident rights. Basic nursing skill information is explained to prepare you to take care of the resident's needs. These needs include measuring vital signs, measuring height and weight, caring for the resident's environment, recognizing abnormal signs and symptoms of common diseases and conditions, and caring for residents when death is near.

Personal care skills for the resident are highlighted in this text. The contents include bathing, grooming, dressing, toileting, eating, and drinking. Skin care techniques, transfers, resident positioning, and turning skills are also included in this section.

Mental health and social service needs of residents are explained in the mental health section. Resident behaviors are discussed and ways to respond to these behaviors are explained. The elderly resident is also discussed.

Care measures for residents with cognitive or mental impairments such as Alzheimer's disease are presented. These measures include communication and behavior methods. Basic restorative procedures are presented to assist you in increasing the resident's level of functioning in daily activities. These include working with the resident on self-care, using assistive devices for ambulation and self-care, performing range-of-motion exercises, using bowel and bladder programs, and using orthotic and prosthetic devices.

Resident rights—the rights to privacy, to choice, to confidentiality, to personal belongings, to resolve grievances and disputes, and the right to freedom from restraints or abuse—are discussed.

Illustrations and pictures enhance the material presented. This text contains the information needed to prepare you for the important job of caring for residents in a nursing facility.

Stephanie Vaughn
Sheila A. Sorrentino

CONTENTS _____

Introduction: Nurse Aide Training and Competency Evaluation, 1

1   Communication and Interpersonal Skills for the Nurse Aide, 3

2   Infection Control, 21

3   Safety and Emergency Procedures, 31

4   Promoting Residents' Adjustment, Independence, and Rights, 43

5   Respecting Residents' Rights, 49

6   Vital Signs, 55

7   Admission and Discharge Processes, 75

8   Caring for the Resident's Environment, 79

9   Recognizing Abnormal Signs and Symptoms of Common Diseases, 97

10 Caring for the Resident When Death is Near, 129

11 Bathing, Grooming, and Dressing, 139

12 Toileting, 159

13 Feeding Techniques, 187

14 Skin Care, 207

15 Transfers and Body Mechanics, 215

16 Mental Health and Social Service Needs, 233

17 Care of Cognitively Impaired Residents, 243

18 Basic Restorative Services, 251

19 Residents' Rights, 273

Glossary, 279

**OBRA Nurse Aide
Skills Manual**

Nurse Aide Training
and Competency Evaluation

The care given by nurse aides is important to the health and welfare of residents in long-term care facilities. Safe, effective, and quality care is essential to protect residents from harm. This is why nurse aide training is required by law in all states. The laws require that individuals learn basic nursing knowledge and skills for employment as nurse aides.

In 1987 the Congress of the United States passed the Omnibus Budget Reconciliation Act (OBRA). This law applies to all states. Its purpose is to improve the quality of care given to residents of nursing facilities by requiring education and competency evaluation for all nurse aides they employ. The requirement ensures that nurse aides have the knowledge and skills to give safe and effective care.

THE TRAINING PROGRAM

Every state must now have a nurse aide training and competency evaluation program. The training program must include at least 75 hours of instruction. Sixteen of the hours must be supervised practical training in a laboratory or clinical setting. The student must perform nursing care and procedures on another individual. This practical training (also called a clinical practicum or clinical experience) is supervised by a nurse. Usually the nurse is the course instructor.

The training program teaches the knowledge and skills needed by nurse aides to perform their roles and responsibilities. Areas to be studied include communication, infection control, safety and emergency procedures, residents' rights, basic nursing skills, personal care skills, feeding techniques, and skin care. Students learn how to transfer, position, turn, dress, and ambulate residents and how to perform range-of-motion exercises. They learn the signs and symptoms of common diseases and conditions and how to care for cognitively impaired residents (those who have problems with thinking and memory).

The competency evaluation program involves a written test and a skills test. Preparation for the competency evaluation begins the first day of your training program. You will learn the basic nursing content areas and the skills for giving safe, quality care. The written and skills competency evaluations are taken after you com-

1

plete the training program. Your instructor or supervisor can help you determine where to take the tests and to complete the required application form. There is also a fee for the competency evaluation, which must be sent with your application. You will be notified where to go and the time of the tests after your application has been processed.

The nurse aide is given a registration number after successfully completing the competency evaluation. This number is given by the state in which the nurse aide took the tests. If unsuccessful, an individual may retake the competency evaluation. OBRA requires that individuals be given three tries to be successful.

NURSE AIDE REGISTRY

OBRA requires each state to establish a registry of nurse aides who have successfully completed a training and competency evaluation program. The registry contains the following information about each nurse aide: name; last known address; registration number and expiration date; date of birth; last known employer; date of hire; date of termination; date the competency evaluation was passed; information regarding any finding of abuse, neglect or dishonest use of property; and date and outcome of any hearings, if applicable. All information remains in the registry for at least 5 years.

OTHER OBRA REQUIREMENTS

OBRA also requires retraining and a new competency evaluation program for nurse aides who have not worked for 2 consecutive years. This is to ensure that you have *current* knowledge and skills to give safe care. It does not matter how long you worked as a nurse aide. What matters is how long you did not work.

Regular in-service education and performance reviews are other OBRA requirements. Nursing facilities must offer regular education programs to nurse aides. The work of each nurse aide must also be regularly evaluated. These are ways to help ensure that nurse aides have the knowledge and skills to give safe, effective care.

CHAPTER 1

Communication and Interpersonal Skills for the Nurse Aide

Objectives

Describe the qualities and characteristics of a successful nurse aide

Identify good health and personal hygiene practices

Describe major areas of responsibility of a nurse aide

Identify information which can be collected about a resident using sight, hearing, touch, and smell

List information which should always be included when reporting to a nurse

List basic rules for recording

Discuss the importance of promoting resident rights

Describe the ethical behavior of the nurse aide

Explain how you can prevent negligent acts

Identify the elements needed for effective communication

Describe how nurse aides use verbal and nonverbal communication

Identify six communication barriers

Explain the purpose, parts, and information found in a resident's record

Describe the legal and ethical responsibilities of nurse aides who have access to resident records

Describe the purpose of the resident care plan and the Kardex; nursing process

QUALITIES AND CHARACTERISTICS OF A NURSE AIDE

Caring about others is a common trait among the health team. Caring enough to want to make the life of a person happier, easier, or less painful is an essential characteristic of a nurse aide. There are traits, attitudes, and manners that allow one to perform a job well. These are called "qualities and characteristics."

3

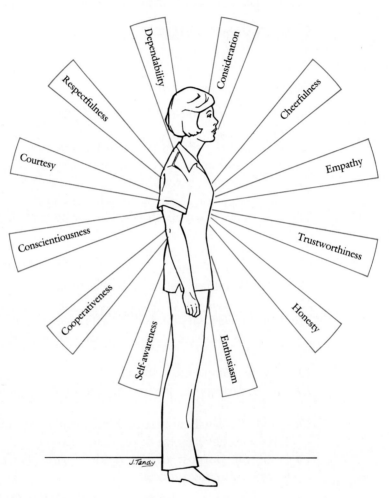

Fig. 1-1 The qualities and characteristics of a successful nurse aide. *(From Sorrentino SA: Mosby's textbook for nursing assistants, ed 3, St Louis, 1992, Mosby–Year Book.)*

Besides caring, the following qualities and characteristics are necessary for you to function effectively (Fig. 1-1).

1. *Dependability.* The residents and members of the nursing team rely on you to report to work on time when scheduled. They also depend on you to perform duties and tasks as assigned, as well as keeping obligations and promises.
2. *Consideration.* You need to be considerate of the resident's physical and personal feelings. Residents should be treated gently and with kindness.
3. *Cheerfulness.* You need to greet and converse with the resident and others in a pleasant manner. You cannot be moody, bad tempered, sarcastic, or unhappy when caring for residents.
4. *Empathy.* Empathy is the ability to see things from the resident's point of view—to put yourself in the resident's position. How would you feel if you had the resident's problems?
5. *Trustworthiness.* Residents and co-workers have placed their confidence in you. They believe you will keep information confidential and not gossip about residents, co-workers, physicians, or members of the health team.
6. *Respectfulness.* Residents have rights, values, beliefs, and feelings. Although these may not be the same as yours, you must not criticize or condemn the resident. The patient is treated with respect and dignity at all times. You must also show respect for supervisors and co-workers.
7. *Courtesy.* You need to be polite and courteous to residents, families, visitors, and co-workers. People are addressed by title and name (for example, "Mrs. Johnson" or "Dr. Wilson"). Other courteous acts include explaining what is going to be done before performing a procedure, saying "please" or "thank you", and not interrupting others unnecessarily.
8. *Conscientiousness.* You must be careful, alert, and exact in following orders and instructions. You must give thorough care with knowledge and skill, and give your best effort.
9. *Honesty.* You must be truthful, sincere, genuine, and show a true interest in the resident. The amount and kind of care given, observations, and errors are reported truthfully and accurately.
10. *Cooperation.* You must be willing to help and work with others. Cooperation is shown by the ability to get along well with others and by taking an "extra step" during busy and stressful times.
11. *Enthusiasm.* Enthusiasm is shown by being excited, interested, and eager about your work. What you are doing is important. If you are enthusiastic, you will want to gain more self-confidence, skill, and knowledge.
12. *Self-awareness.* Being self-aware means that you know your feelings, strengths, and weaknesses. You need to understand yourself before you can understand residents.

PERSONAL HEALTH, HYGIENE, AND APPEARANCE

Residents, families, and visitors expect the health team to be a good example of healthy habits. Your personal health, appearance, and hygiene deserve careful attention. It's important to eat a balanced diet from the four food groups (dairy, fish and meat, fruits and vegetables, and bread) each day. Adequate sleep and rest are also needed to do your job well and stay healthy. Regular exercise helps you feel better physically and more alert mentally.

Smoking has been linked to lung cancer and circulatory disorders. If you smoke, remember that it can be offensive to others. Smoke only in areas where it is allowed. Smoke odors stay on hands, clothing, and hair. Therefore, handwashing and good personal hygiene are essential. Wash your hands immediately after smoking and before giving resident care.

Drugs and alcohol have an undesirable effect on your mind and body and will affect your ability to work effectively. Working under the influence of drugs and alcohol places your residents in danger. You should never report to work under the influence of drugs of alcohol. The safety of your residents, co-workers, and yourself must be considered.

Preventing offensive body and breath odors is important. You should bathe daily, use a deodorant or antiperspirant, brush your teeth after meals, and use a mouthwash regularly. Your hair should be clean and styled in an attractive, simple way. Fingernails should be clean, short, and neatly shaped.

Jewelry should not be worn while on duty. Most facilities let employees wear wedding rings. Engagement rings may be allowed. Large rings and bracelets can scratch residents. Necklaces, bracelets, and earrings can easily be pulled off by confused or combative residents, causing physical injury to you.

FUNCTIONS AND RESPONSIBILITIES

Nurse aide functions and responsibilities vary among health care facilities. *Responsibility* is a duty or obligation to perform an act and being able to answer for one's actions.

Nurse aides perform functions and procedures relating to personal hygiene, safety, nutrition, exercise, and elimination needs. Related functions include lifting and moving patients, observing the patient, helping promote physical comfort, and collecting specimens. Nurse aides may also assist with the admission or discharge of residents and measure temperatures, pulses, respirations, and blood pressures.

Your training may prepare you to perform certain procedures. However, your employer may not allow nurse aides to perform them. Other facilities may teach nurse aides perform procedures and tasks that they did not learn previously.

Functions

There are certain functions, procedures, and tasks that nurse aides never perform. It is extremely important that you understand what procedures you *cannot* do as a nurse aide. Never give medications by any route; never insert tubes or objects into body openings; never take orders from a physician; never perform procedures that require sterile technique; never tell the resident or family the resident's diagnosis or treatment plan; never diagnose or prescribe treatments or medications for residents; never supervise other nurse aides; and immediately tell the nurse about any order or request that is beyond the scope of nurse aides so that the resident's needs can be met.

Responsibilities

I. Resident care
   A. Treat residents with respect at all times; promote and respect residents' rights.
   B. Observe and recognize signs of common conditions.
   C. Measure vital signs, height, and weight.
   D. Provide personal care such as baths, showers, oral hygiene, skin care, hair care, fingernail and toenail care, monitoring fluid intake and output, toileting care, etc.
   E. Assist the male resident to shave daily.
   F. Assist in serving and feeding residents.
   G. Distribute fresh drinking water each shift.
   H. Use safety measures for residents and self when using body mechanics, side rails, collapsible tubs, etc.
   I. Assist with restorative nursing procedures. These may include:
      1. Good body alignment
      2. Bed positioning
      3. Range-of-motion (ROM) exercises
      4. Transferring patients with use of a gait belt
      5. Other procedures
   J. Follow the bowel or bladder training program established for a resident.
   K. Assist the resident to the bathroom as necessary.
   L. Encourage and assist the resident to attend all therapies and programs ordered by the doctor (for example, physical therapy).
   M. Assist the resident to follow through and practice activities or exercises learned in the therapy program.
   N. Assist in 24-hour Reality Orientation.
   O. Plan and organizes care so residents can attend activities or therapies as scheduled.

P. Assist in transferring residents to activity programs.
Q. Make regular rounds to all residents and provides necessary care.
R. Answer call lights promptly and provide or obtain the necessary care.
S. Observe and report unusual symptoms, changes, accidents, and injuries to the charge nurse.
T. Participate in the residents' care conferences.
U. Report to the charge nurse before going off duty.
V. Perform other duties as directed by the supervisor.

II. Environmental
A. Make beds and clean units daily as assigned by the charge nurse.
B. Care for linen and other laundry according to procedure.
C. Follow established cleaning schedule for drawers, closets, utility rooms, and nurses' station.
D. Clean and care for equipment and utensils as assigned by the charge nurse.

COMMUNICATION

Health team members must communicate with each other for coordinated and effective resident care. Information must be shared about what has been done and what needs to be done for the resident. Information about the resident's response to treatment must also be shared.

Communication is the exchange of information—a message sent is received and interpreted by the intended person(s). For communication to be effective, words must have the same meaning for the sender and receiver of the message. The words "small", "moderate", and "large" are often used in health care. Unfortunately, they mean different things to different people. Is small the size of a dime or a half dollar? In health care, differences in meaning can have serious consequences. Avoid words that might have more than one meaning.

Using words familiar to people you communicate with is important. You will learn medical terminology as you study and gain experience as a nurse aide. If a nurse or health team member uses an unfamiliar term, ask for an explanation. If you do not understand the message sent to you, communication will not have occurred. Likewise, remember not to use terms that are unfamiliar to residents.

Try to be brief and concise when communicating. Do not add unrelated or nonessential information. You must stay on the subject, avoid wandering in thought, and not get wordy. Being brief and concise reduces the possibility of omitting important details.

Information should be presented in a logical and orderly manner. Organize your thoughts so that you can present them logically and in sequence. Think about what happened step by step and present the information to the nurse in that way.

You need to present facts and be specific when giving information. The receiver should have a clear picture of what you are communicating.

Nonverbal communication or body language is messages given without the use of words, or used with verbal communication to enhance or add meaning to what is being said. Examples of body language include hand gestures and facial expressions.

Communicating with the resident

Several elements are necessary for effective communication between you and the resident. First, you must understand and respect your resident as a person. Second, the resident must be viewed as more than a disease or illness; the resident is a physical, psychological, social, and spiritual human. Third, you need to recognize and respect the resident's rights. Finally, you must accept and respect the resident's religion and culture.

Verbal and nonverbal methods of communication are used when relating to residents. You need to understand how to use both methods for effective communication.

Verbal communication. Words are used in *verbal communication*. They may be spoken or written. Verbal communication is used to talk to residents, to find out how they are feeling physically and emotionally, and to share information with them.

Most verbal communication involves words. You need to control the loudness and tone of your voice, speak clearly and distinctly, and avoid using slang or vulgar words. Shouting, whispering, and mumbling cause poor communication.

Written words are used when residents cannot speak or hear. If a resident cannot speak, provide a way for the resident to send messages. A Magic Slate, paper and

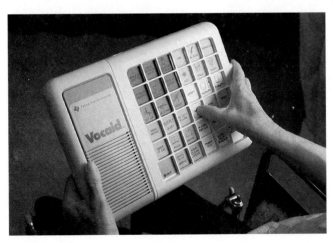

Fig. 1-2 Resident using an electronic talking aid. (*From Sorrentino SA:* Mosby's textbook for nursing assistants, *ed 3, St Louis, 1992, Mosby–Year Book.*)

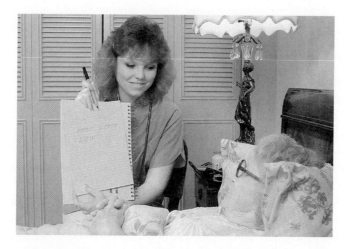

Fig. 1-3 Nurse aide writing a note to a resident with hearing deficit. (*From Sorrentino SA: Mosby's textbook for nursing assistants, ed 3, St Louis, 1992, Mosby–Year Book.*)

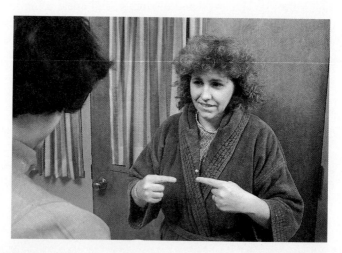

Fig. 1-4 Resident using sign language to communicate. (*From Sorrentino SA: Mosby's textbook for nursing assistants, ed 3, St Louis, 1992, Mosby–Year Book.*)

pencil, or an electronic talking aid (Fig. 1-2) can be used. Write messages to communicate with deaf residents or those with severe hearing problems (Fig. 1-3). Deaf residents may use sign language to communicate (Fig. 1-4).

Communication between you and the resident should be kept on a professional level. You should not become personally involved or develop friendships with residents.

Nonverbal communication. *Nonverbal communication* does not involve words. Gestures, facial expressions, posture, body movements, touch, and smell are examples of how messages can be sent and received without words. Nonverbal messages are considered to be a true reflection of a person's feelings. They are usually involuntary and difficult to control. A resident may say one thing but act in a different way. Therefore, you need to watch the resident's eyes, the way hands are held or moved, gestures, posture, and other actions—body language. Body language also can add meaning to what is being said.

Barriers to effective communication. Communication may fail to occur for many reasons. You and the resident must use and understand the same language. If not, messages will not be accurately shared.

Changing the subject is another barrier to communication. Either you or the resident may change the subject when the topic being discussed is uncomfortable. Avoid changing the subject whenever possible.

Let residents express their feelings and concerns without adding your opinion, making a judgment, or jumping to conclusions.

Some nurse aides talk a lot to residents. Too much talking is usually due to nervousness and being uncomfortable with silence. Silences have meaning. Acceptance, rejection, fear, or the need for quiet and time to think may be conveyed by silence.

Listening is very important for effective communication. Communication will be blocked if you fail to listen to your residents with interest and sincerity. Do not pretend to listen. This causes the wrong responses to the resident and conveys a lack of interest and caring. You may also miss important complaints of pain, discomfort, or other abnormal sensations that must be reported to the nurse.

Answers such as "Don't worry", "Everything will be okay", and "Your doctor knows best" block communication. These make residents feel that their concerns, feelings, and fears are being ridiculed and are not important to you or the nursing team.

Reporting and recording observations

Reporting and recording are ways in which communication takes place among health team members. Both are accounts of what has been done for and observed about the patient. *Reporting* is the verbal account of resident care and observations. *Recording* or *charting* is the written account.

BASIC OBSERVATIONS OF THE RESIDENT

Ability to respond
- Is the resident easy or difficult to arouse?
- Is the resident able to give his or her name, the time, and the location when asked?
- Can the resident identify others accurately?
- Can the resident answer questions correctly?
- Can the resident speak clearly?
- Are instructions followed appropriately?
- Is the resident calm, restless, or excited?
- Is the resident conversing, quiet, or talking a lot?

Movement
- Can the resident squeeze your fingers with each hand?
- Can the resident move arms and legs?
- Are the resident's movements shaky or jerky?

Pain or discomfort
- Where is the pain located? (Ask resident to point to the pain.)
- Does the pain go anywhere else?
- How long does the pain last?
- How does the resident describe the pain?

Sharp	Aching
Severe	Comes and
Knifelike	goes
Dull	Depends on
Burning	position

Pain or Discomfort—cont'd
- Has medication been given?
- Did medication help relieve the pain? Is pain still present?
- Is the resident able to sleep and rest?
- What is the position of comfort?

Skin
- Is the skin pale or flushed?
- Is the skin cool, warm, or hot?
- Is the skin moist or dry?
- What color are the lips and nails?
- Are there any sores or reddened areas?

Eyes, ears, nose, and mouth
- Is there drainage from the eyes?
- Are the eyelids closed?
- Are the eyes reddened?
- Does the resident complain of spots, flashes, or blurring?
- Is the resident sensitive to bright lights?
- Is there drainage from the ears?
- Can the resident hear? Is repeating necessary? Are questions answered appropriately?
- Is there drainage from the nose?
- Can the resident breathe through the nose?
- Is there breath odor?
- Does the resident complain of a bad taste in the mouth?

Respirations

- Do both sides of the resident's chest rise and fall with respirations?
- Is there noisy breathing?
- Is there difficulty breathing?
- What is the amount and color of sputum?
- What is the frequency of the resident's cough? Is it dry or productive?

Bowels and bladder

- Is the abdomen firm or soft?
- Does the resident complain of gas?
- What is the amount, color, and consistency of bowel movements?
- Does the resident have pain or difficulty while urinating?
- What is the amount of urine?
- What is the frequency of urination?
- What is the frequency of bowel movements?

Appetite

- Does the resident like the diet?
- How much of the food on the tray is eaten?
- What are the resident's food preferences?
- How much liquid was taken?
- What are the resident's liquid preferences?
- How often does the resident drink liquids?
- Is the resident experiencing nausea?
- What is the amount and color of material vomited?
- Does the resident have hiccups?
- Is the resident belching?

Activities of daily living

- Can the resident perform personal care without help?
    Bathing
    Brushing teeth
    Combing and brushing hair
    Shaving
- Does the resident use a toilet, commode, bedpan, or urinal?
- Is the resident able to feed self?
- Is the resident able to walk?
- What amount and kind of assistance is needed?

Observations. *Observation* is using the senses of sight, hearing, touch, and smell to collect information. You will observe such things as the way the patient is lying, sitting, or walking. You will also observe if the resident's skin is flushed or pale, and if there are reddened or swollen body areas. You will listen to the resident breathe, talk, and cough, and you will use a stethoscope to listen to the heartbeat. By touching the resident you can collect information about skin temperature and feel if the skin is moist or dry. You will also use touch to take the resident's pulse. The sense of smell is used to detect body, wound, and breath odors or unusual odors from urine and bowel movements.

Information observed about a resident is called objective data. *Objective data (signs)* are those things you can see, hear, feel, or smell. You can feel a pulse and you can see what a resident has vomited. However, you cannot feel or see the resident's pain or nausea. The things a resident tells you about but that you cannot observe through your senses are *subjective data (symptoms)*. Opinions are also considered subjective, therefore it is important to focus on signs that you observe (objective) and the resident's responses.

There are many other things you will observe about the residents. More specific observations are discussed as they relate to procedures and resident care presented throughout this book. The box on pp. 12-13 lists the basic observations you need to make and report to the nurse.

You should make notes of your observations. They will be valuable later when you report to the nurse. Carry a note pad and pen in your pocket so you can note your observations at the time they are made.

Reporting. The nurse aide reports about resident care and observations to the nurse. Reports must be prompt, thorough, and accurate. Always give the nurse the resident's name and the time your observations were made or the care that was given. Only report those things that you observed or did yourself. Use your written notes to give the report in a specific, concise, and descriptive manner.

The nurse gives a report at the end of the shift to nursing personnel of the oncoming shift (end-of-shift report). Information is shared about the care that has been given and the care that needs to be given to residents. Information about the resident's condition is also included. Some facilities require that all members of the nursing team hear the end-of-shift report as they come on duty. Others require that nurse aides perform routine tasks while RNs and LPNs hear the report.

Recording. If allowed to record on the resident's chart, you have an even greater responsibility to communicate clearly and thoroughly. You should follow these basic rules when recording:

1. Always use ink.
2. Include the date and time a recording is made.
3. Make sure writing is legible and neat.

4. Only use abbreviations approved by the facility in which you work.
5. Use correct spelling, grammar, and punctuation.
6. Never erase if you make an error. Cross out the incorrect part, write "error" over it, and rewrite the part.
7. Sign all entries with your name and title as required by facility policy (for example, Joan Smith, NA).
8. Do not skip lines. Draw a line through the blank space of a partially completed line to prevent others from recording in a space with your signature.
9. Make sure each form on which you are writing is stamped with the resident's name and other identifying information.
10. Record only what you have observed and done yourself.
11. Never chart a procedure or treatment until it has been completed.
12. Be accurate, concise, and factual. Do not record judgments or interpretations.
13. Record in a logical manner, listing observations, procedures and treatments in the order in which they occurred.
14. Be descriptive. Avoid terms that have more than one meaning.
15. Use the resident's exact words whenever possible. Use quotation marks to show that the statement is a direct quote.

PROMOTING RESIDENT RIGHTS

The resident is the most important person in the health-care facility. Age, religion, nationality, education, occupation, and life-style are some factors that make each resident unique. The resident must be treated as a human and as a person who is valuable, important, and special. The resident must also be treated as an individual who can think, act, and make decisions.

You will care for many residents. Remember that each one is a person. You need to understand their fears, needs, and rights.

Resident's rights have an ethical and legal basis. The right to privacy and informed consent are basic and important rights.

The Omnibus Budget Reconciliation Act (OBRA) of 1987 outlines the rights of residents in nursing facilities. The rights include right to privacy; personal choice; right to voice concerns and have disputes resolved; right to keep and use personal possessions; and freedom from abuse, mistreatment, neglect, and restraints.

ETHICAL AND LEGAL CONSIDERATIONS

As a nurse aide, you will often be in situations in which you must decide what you should or should not do, or what you can or cannot do. These questions may involve ethical considerations, or they may be of a legal nature.

Ethics

Ethics is concerned with what is right and wrong conduct. It involves morals and making choices or judgments about what should or should not be done. An ethical person behaves and acts in the right way.

Professional groups may have a code of ethics. The code consists of rules or standards of conduct that members of the group follow. The American Nurses' Association has a code of ethics for RNs, and the National Federation of Licensed Practical Nurses has a code of ethics for LPNs. You should develop your personal code of ethics. Consider the following rules of conduct for nurse aides.

1. Respect each resident as an individual.
2. Perform no act that is not within the legal scope of the nurse aide.
3. Perform no act for which you have not been adequately prepared.
4. Take no drug without the prescription and supervision of a physician.
5. Carry out the directions and instructions of the nurse to your best possible ability.
6. Be loyal to your employer and co-workers.
7. Be a responsible citizen at all times.
8. Recognize the limits of your role and knowledge.
9. Keep resident information confidential.
10. Consider the resident's needs to be more important than your own.

Legal considerations

Legal considerations relate to laws. A *law* is a rule of conduct made by a government body such as Congress or a state legislature. Laws protect the public welfare and are enforced by the government.

Criminal laws are concerned with offenses against the public and against society in general. A violation of a criminal law is called a *crime*. A person found guilty of a crime will be fined or sent to prison. Murder, robbery, rape, and kidnapping are examples of crimes.

Civil laws are concerned with the relationships between people. Examples of civil laws are those that pertain to contracts and nursing practice. An individual guilty of breaking a civil law usually has to pay a sum of money to the injured person.

Negligence is an unintentional wrong. The person fails to act in a reasonable and careful manner and thereby causes harm to the person or property of another. The negligent person failed to do what a reasonable and careful person would have done, or did what a reasonable and careful person would not have done. The negligent person may have to pay damages (for example, a sum of money) to the injured party.

Malpractice refers to negligence by professionals. A person is considered to be a professional because of training, education, and the type of service provided. Nurses, doctors, lawyers, and pharmacists are examples of professional people.

Some common negligent acts committed by nurse aides are:

1. The side rails are left down on the bed of a confused resident. The resident falls out of bed and breaks a hip.
2. A resident is burned because a nurse aide applied a warm water bottle that was too hot.
3. A resident's dentures break after being dropped by the nurse aide.

As a nurse aide you are legally responsible *(liable)* for your actions. What you do or do not do can lead to a lawsuit if harm results to the person or property of a resident. At times a nurse may direct you to do something that is beyond the legal scope of your role or for which you have not been prepared. The nurse will be held liable as your supervisor, but in no way are you relieved of personal liability. *You are responsible for your actions.*

The resident must give consent for any procedure, treatment, or other act that involves touching the body. The resident has the right to withdraw consent at any time.

Consent is more than the resident's verbal approval or signature on a form. For the resident's consent to be valid, it must be *informed* consent. Informed consent recognizes a person's right to decide what will be done to his or her body and who will be allowed to touch his or her body. Consent is considered to be informed when the resident clearly understands the reason for a treatment, what will be done, how it will be done, who will do it, and the expected outcomes. The resident also must understand the treatment alternatives and the consequences of not having the treatment. The responsibility of informing the resident rests with the physician.

Every person has the right not to have their name, photograph, or private affairs exposed or made public without having given consent. A violation of this right is an *invasion of privacy*. You must treat residents with respect and ensure their privacy. Only health workers involved in the resident's care should see, handle, or examine the resident's body. You can ensure the resident's right to privacy by keeping the resident covered, screen the resident when providing care, and do not discuss a resident's condition with anyone except the charge nurse.

RESIDENT'S RECORD

The *resident's record (chart)* is a written account of the resident's treatment and care. The primary purpose of the resident's record is to provide a way for the health team to communicate information about the resident. The record is permanent and can be retrieved many years later if the resident's health history is needed. The record is a legal document. It can be used in a court of law as evidence of the resident's problems, treatment, and care.

The record has many forms organized into sections for easy use. It includes the resident's history of physical examinations, doctor's orders, and doctor's progress notes. Also included are the graphic sheet, x-ray reports, IV therapy record, respiratory therapy record, consultation reports, and admission sheet. Each page must be stamped with the resident's name, room number, and other identifying information. This helps prevent errors and the wrong placement of records.

Members of the health team record information on the forms for their department and service. The information is then available to other health team members who need to know what care has been provided.

Some facilities do not allow nurse aides to write in resident records. They feel that this is a nurse's responsibility. Other facilities rely on nurse aides to record observations on care.

Usually, all professional health workers involved in the resident's care have access to the resident's record. Those not directly involved usually are not allowed to review the record. Some facilities do not let nurse aides read the charts. In such instances the nurse shares necessary information with nurse aides.

If you have access to resident records, you have an ethical and legal responsibility to keep the information confidential. Also remember that only members of the health team involved in the resident's care need to read the chart.

The following parts of the resident's record relate to your work as a nurse aide: admission sheet, graphic sheet (for vital signs, intake and output), nurse's notes and flow sheets.

NURSING CARE PLAN

The *nursing care plan* is a written guide that gives direction about the care a resident should receive. The plan consists of resident problems identified by the nurse and the actions nursing personnel will take to help solve them. The nurse responsible for the resident's care develops the care plan. Some nurses welcome suggestions from nurse aides when developing nursing care plans.

A care plan is developed for each resident. You can use the nursing care plan as a guide to care of a resident.

Forms for nursing care plans vary in each facility. Often the care plan is included in the resident's record or in a Kardex.

KARDEX

The *Kardex* is a type of card file used in health care facilities. There is a card for each resident which contains some of the information found in the resident's record.

Diet:			

Activities:	Bath:	Travel:	Position:
___ Complete bed rest ___ Bed rest ___ Bathroom privileges ✓ Up ad lib	___ Bed bath ___ Partial ✓ Bathe self ___ Tub ___ Shower	___ Wheelchair ___ Stretcher ✓ Ambulatory ___ Walker ___ Cane ___ Crutches	

Side rails:	Oxygen:	Special equipment:
___ Constantly ___ Nights only ✓ Side rail release	___ Liters per minute ___ PRN ___ Constantly ___ Tent ___ Catheter ___ Mask ___ Cannula	

Prosthesis:	Special privileges:	
___ Dentures ✓ Eye glasses ___ Contact lenses ___ Hearing aid ___ Limb ___ Other	May shampoo hair as desired	Allergies: None known

Date	Medications	Date	Treatments
8/21	Tagamet 300 mg qid — 9-1-5-9 — po	8/21	Vital signs — qid
8/21	Mylanta 10 ml po 90 min pc + HS		Fluids
		8/21	Intake and output
		8/21	Hematest stools for occult blood
8/22	HS Med Dalmane 30 mg po		
PRN 8/22	Tylenol tabs 2 po q4h — headache		IVs
		8/21	D5W 1000 ml q 8h

Room	Name	Age	Diagnosis	Doctor
333-1	Bailey, Laura	46	Duodenal ulcer	J. Wilson

Fig. 1-5 A sample Kardex. *(From Sorrentino SA:* Mosby's textbook for nursing assistants, *ed 3, St Louis, 1992, Mosby–Year Book.)*

The Kardex is basically a summary of the current medications and treatments ordered by the doctor, the resident's current diagnosis, routine care measures, and special equipment needs. The Kardex is a quick and easy source of resident information (Fig. 1-5).

SUMMARY

This chapter discussed the characteristics and the role of the nurse aide. Ethical and legal considerations about the job were presented. Communication among members of the health team is essential for effective and coordinated care of the resident. Communication is verbal or nonverbal. It should be factual, concise, and understandable. Resident records such as the chart, Kardex, and care plan are ways in which health team members communicate with each other.

CHAPTER 2

Infection Control

Objectives

Explain the difference between pathogens and nonpathogens

Identify six things needed by microorganisms to live and grow

Identify the signs and symptoms of an infection

Describe six things needed for an infection to develop

Explain the differences between medical asepsis, disinfection, and sterilization

Describe the practice of medical asepsis, two methods of sterilization, and how to care for equipment and supplies

Explain the purpose of infection precautions and their effects on the resident

Describe universal precautions and the general rules for maintaining them

Infection is a major safety and health hazard. Some infections are minor and cause short illnesses. Others are very serious and can cause death. The health team must protect residents and themselves by preventing the spread of infection.

MICROORGANISMS

A *microorganism* is a small *(micro)* living plant or animal *(organism)* that cannot be seen without a microscope. Microorganisms (microbes) are everywhere. They are in our air, food, mouth, nose, respiratory tract, stomach, intestines, and on the skin. They are in the soil and water, and are found on animals, clothing, and furniture. Some microbes cause infections and are considered harmful. They are called *pathogens*. *Nonpathogens* are microorganisms that do not usually cause an infection.

Types of microorganisms

There are five general types of microorganisms.

1. *Bacteria* are microscopic plant life that multiply rapidly. They consist of a single cell and are often called *germs*.
2. *Fungi* are plants that live on other plants or animals. Mushrooms, yeasts, and molds are common fungi.
3. *Protozoa* are microscopic one-celled animals.
4. *Rickettsiae* are microscopic forms of life found in the tissues of fleas, lice, ticks, and other insects. They are transmitted to humans by insect bites.
5. *Viruses* are very small microscopic organisms that grow in living cells.

Requirements of microorganisms

Microorganisms need a reservoir to live and grow. The *reservoir* or *host* is the environment in which the microorganism lives and grows. The reservoir can be a human, a plant, an animal, soil, food, water, or other material. The microorganism must get *water* and *nourishment* from the reservoir. Most microbes need *oxygen* to live. Others cannot live in the presence of oxygen. A *warm* and *dark* environment is needed. Most microorganisms grow best at body temperature and are destroyed by heat and light.

Normal flora

Normal flora refers to microorganisms that usually live and grow in a certain location. Microbes are found in the respiratory tract, in the intestines, on the skin, and in other sites outside the body. They are nonpathogenic when in or on a natural reservoir. If a nonpathogen is transmitted from its natural location to another site or host, it becomes a pathogen. For example, *Escherichia coli* is a microorganism normally found in the large intestine. If *E. coli* enters the urinary system, it can cause an infection.

INFECTION

An *infection* is a disease state resulting from the invasion and growth of microorganisms in the body. It may be localized in a specific body part or involve the whole body. A person with an infection has certain signs and symptoms. Some or all of the following may be present: fever, pain or tenderness, fatigue, loss of appetite, nausea, vomiting, diarrhea, rash, sores on mucous membranes, redness and swelling of a body part, and discharge or drainage from the infected area. Pathogenic microorganisms can be present without causing an infection. The development of an infection depends on several factors.

The process of infection

For an infection to develop there must be a *source*. The source is a pathogen capable of causing disease. The pathogen must have a *reservoir* where it can grow and multiply. Humans and animals are reservoirs for microbes. If they do not have signs and symptoms of infection, they are *carriers*. Carriers can pass the pathogen on to other people. The pathogen must be able to leave the reservoir. In other words, it must have an *exit*. Exits in the human body are the respiratory, gastrointestinal, urinary, and reproductive tracts; breaks in the skin; and the blood.

A pathogen that has left the reservoir must be *transmitted* to another host. Methods of transmission include direct contact, air, food, water, animals, and insects. Microbes can also be transmitted by eating and drinking utensils, dressings, and equipment for personal care and hygiene (Fig. 2-1). The pathogen must then enter the body through a *portal of entry*. Portals of entry are the same as the exits. Whether or not the pathogen grows and multiplies depends on the *susceptibility of the host*. The human body has a natural ability to protect itself from infection. A person's ability to resist infection is related to age, sex, nutritional status, fatigue, general health, medications, and the presence or absence of other illnesses. (Table 1).

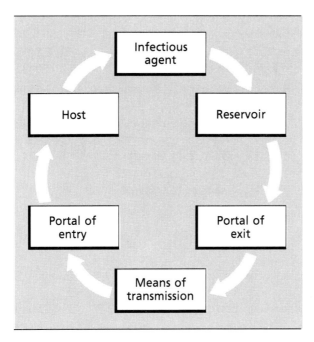

Fig. 2-1 Chain of infection. *(From Potter PA, Perry AG:* Fundamentals of nursing concepts, process, and practice, *ed 2, St Louis, 1989, Mosby–Year Book.)*

Table 1 Common pathogens and some infections or diseases they produce

Organism	Reservoir	Infection or disease
Bacteria		
Staphylococcus aureus	Skin, hair, anterior nares	Wound infection, pneumonia, food poisoning, cellulitis
Streptococcus (beta-hemolytic group A)	Oropharynx, skin, perianal area	"Strep throat," rheumatic fever, scarlet fever, impetigo
Streptococcus (beta-hemolytic group B)	Adult genitalia	Urinary tract infection, wound infection, endometritis
Escherichia coli	Colon	Enteritis
Neisseria gonorrhoeae	Genitourinary tract, rectum, mouth, eye	Gonorrhea, pelvic inflammatory disease, infectious arthritis, conjunctivitis
Viruses		
Herpes simplex 1	Lesions of mouth, skin, blood, excretions	Cold sores, aseptic meningitis, sexually transmitted disease
Hepatitis A	Feces, blood, urine	Infectious hepatitis
Hepatitis B	Feces, blood, all body fluids and excretions	Serum hepatitis
HIV	Blood, semen, and vaginal secretions (also isolated in saliva, tears, urine, and breast milk but not proven to be sources of transmission)	Acquired immunodeficiency syndrome
Fungi		
Candida albicans	Mouth, skin, colon, genital tract	Thrush, dermatitis
Aspergillus	Soil, dust	Aspergillosis
Protozoa		
Plasmodium falciparum	Mosquito	Malaria
Rickettsia		
Rickettsia rickettsii	Wood tick	Rocky Mountain spotted fever

From Perry AG, Potter PA: *Clinical nursing skills and techniques*, ed 2, St Louis, 1990, Mosby–Year Book.

MEDICAL ASEPSIS

Asepsis is the absence of all disease-producing microorganisms (pathogens). Because microbes are everywhere, there must be practices used to achieve asepsis. These practices are known as *medical asepsis* or *clean technique*. Therefore, medical asepsis is the techniques and practices used to prevent the spread of pathogenic microorganisms from one person or place to another person or place. An example of a common medical asepsis practice is washing the hands. Medical asepsis is different from disinfection and sterilization. *Disinfection* is the process in which pathogenic microorganisms are destroyed. *Sterilization* is the process in which *all* microorganisms are destroyed. *Sterile* means the absence of *all* microorganisms, both pathogenic and nonpathogenic.

Contamination is the process by which an object or area becomes unclean. In medical asepsis, an object or area is considered clean when it is free of pathogens. Therefore, the object or area is contaminated if pathogens are present. Likewise, a sterile object or area is contaminated when pathogens or nonpathogens are present.

Handwashing

Handwashing with soap and water is the easiest and a most important way to prevent the spread of infection. The hands are used in almost every resident-care activity. They are easily contaminated and can spread microorganisms if the nurse aide does not practice handwashing before and after giving resident care. To properly wash your hands, you need to follow these rules.

1. Wash your hands under warm, running water.
2. Hand-operated faucets are considered contaminated. Use a paper towel to turn the water off at the end of the handwashing procedure. The paper towel prevents a clean hand from becoming contaminated again. Some facilities consider hand controls to be clean. If hand controls are considered "clean", do not use a paper towel when turning the faucet on and off.
3. Bar soap is held during the entire handwashing procedure. When the procedure is complete, the soap is rinsed under running water. After rinsing, the soap is dropped into the soap dish. Be careful not to touch the soap dish during or after the handwashing procedure. Health care facilities usually have soap dispensers. Bar soap is used in home care.
4. Your hands and forearms are held lower than your elbows throughout the procedure. If your hands and forearms are held up, dirty water can run from the hands to the elbows, contaminating those areas.
5. Attention is given to those areas frequently missed during handwashing: thumbs, knuckles, sides of the hands, little fingers, and underneath the nails. Your hands and wrists should be washed thoroughly by rubbing palms together, rubbing finger tips into palms, and using rotary motion and friction (Fig. 2-2). A nail file or orange stick is used to clean under fingernails.
6. A lotion should be used after handwashing to prevent chapping and drying of the skin.

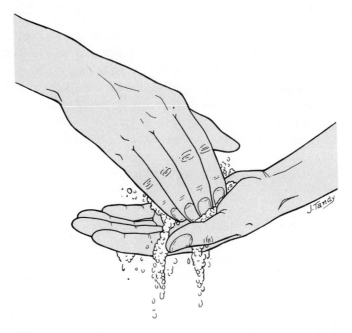

Fig. 2-2 Tips of fingers are rubbed against palm. *(From Sorrentino SA:* Mosby's textbook for nursing assistants, *ed 3, St Louis, 1992, Mosby–Year Book.)*

Care of supplies and equipment. Most facilities have a central supply department that buys, disinfects, sterilizes, and distributes equipment. Much of the equipment is disposable. Disposable equipment is used once for an individual and then discarded. However, some disposable equipment can be used several times by one resident. Examples include disposable bedpans, urinals, wash basins, thermometers, water pitchers, and drinking cups. Disposable equipment helps reduce the spread of infection.

Larger and more expensive equipment is usually not disposable. It must be disinfected or sterilized before being used again by any resident. Prior to disinfection or sterilization, equipment is cleaned. Cleaning reduces the number of microbes to be destroyed and removes organic material. Organic material includes blood, pus, drainage from wounds, and body secretions or excretions. You should use the following general guidelines when cleaning equipment.

1. Rinse the item in cold water first to remove organic material. Heat causes organic material to become thick, sticky, and hard to remove.
2. Use soap and hot water to wash the item.
3. Use a brush if necessary.

4. Rinse and dry the item.
5. Disinfect or sterilize the item.
6. Disinfect equipment used in the cleaning procedure.

Disinfection

Disinfection is the process in which pathogenic microorganisms are destroyed. However, disinfection does not destroy spores. *Spores* are bacteria protected by a hard shell that forms around the microorganism. Spores are killed only by extremely high temperatures. Disinfection methods usually do not destroy all spores.

Boiling water is a simple, inexpensive method of disinfection. It can be done in the home. Small items can be disinfected by placing them in boiling water for at least 15 minutes.

Chemical disinfectants are usually used for housekeeping and cleaning instruments and equipment. They are used to clean commodes, wheelchairs, stretchers, and furniture in the resident's room after a resident has been discharged. There are many types of chemical disinfectants. You should wear waterproof gloves when using a disinfectant to prevent skin irritation. Some chemical disinfectants may have special precautions when being used or stored. Ask the nurse about procedures for a specific disinfectant.

Sterilization

Sterilization procedures destroy all pathogens, nonpathogens, and spores. Extremely high temperatures are used. As stated earlier, microbes grow best at body temperature and are destroyed by heat.

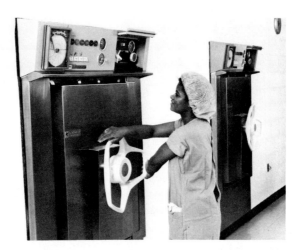

Fig. 2-3 An autoclave. *(From Sorrentino SA:* Mosby's textbook for nursing assistants, *ed 3, St Louis, 1992, Mosby–Year Book.)*

You may learn to sterilize equipment when *steam under pressure* is the method used. An *autoclave* (Fig. 2-3) is a pressure steam sterilizer used to sterilize metal objects such as basins, bedpans, and urinals. Plastic and rubber items, which are destroyed by high temperatures, are not placed in autoclaves. Pressure cookers used to prepare food can sterilize objects in the home. Steam under pressure usually sterilizes objects in 30 to 45 minutes.

Radiation, liquid chemicals, and a chemical gas may be used for sterilizing. Nurse aides are generally not responsible for using these methods.

Other aseptic measures

You should practice additional aseptic measures to prevent the spread of infection and microorganisms. These measures can also be used in the home and in everyday activities.

1. Hold equipment and linens away from your uniform.
2. Avoid shaking linens and other equipment and use a damp cloth to dust furniture. These actions help prevent the movement of dust.
3. Clean from the cleanest area to the dirtiest. This prevents soiling a clean area.
4. Clean away from your body and uniform. If you dust, brush, or wipe toward yourself, microorganisms will be transmitted to your skin, hair, and uniform.
5. Pour contaminated liquids directly into sinks or toilets. Avoid splashing onto other areas.
6. Avoid sitting on a resident's bed. You will pick up microorganisms and transfer them to the next surface that you sit on.
7. Do not take equipment or linen from one resident's room to use for another resident. Even if the item has not been used, do not take it from one room to another.

INFECTIONS PRECAUTIONS

Sometimes other measures are needed to prevent the spread of microorganisms. *Infection precautions* prevent the spread of pathogens from one area to another. Barriers are set up that prevent the escape of pathogens. The pathogens are kept within a specific area, usually the resident's room. The Centers for Disease Control (CDC) in Atlanta, Georgia have developed guidelines for infection precautions. Those guidelines are included in this section.

Instead of "infection precautions", you may hear the phrase "isolation techniques". The word "isolation" implies separating the resident from others. The pathogen is undesirable, not the resident. Therefore, CDC guidelines now use the phrase "infection precautions". However, "isolation" and "isolation techniques" are still used in nursing facilities when describing infection precautions.

Purpose. Infection precautions prevent the spread of a *communicable* or *contagious disease*. Communicable diseases are caused by pathogens that are spread easily. Common communicable diseases are measles, mumps, chicken pox, syphilis, gonorrhea, and acquired immunodeficiency syndrome (AIDS). Residents may have respiratory, wound, skin, gastrointestinal, or blood infections that are highly contagious. Infection precautions are indicated for these residents. Pathogens causing these infections are kept in a specific area.

Infection precautions are sometimes used to protect a resident. Age, weakness, illness, and certain medications make some residents very susceptible to infection. Their ability to fight an infection is reduced. If an infection develops, the consequences can be quite severe.

Clean versus dirty

Infection precautions are based on an understanding of "clean" and "dirty." "Clean" refers to those areas or objects that are uncontaminated. Uncontaminated areas are free of pathogens. Areas or objects considered "dirty" are those that are contaminated. If a clean area of an object comes in contact with something dirty, the object or area that was clean is now considered dirty. Clean and dirty also depend on the way in which the pathogen is spread.

Universal precautions

Universal precautions were issued by the CDC in 1987. They were developed to prevent the spread of AIDS. The virus that causes AIDS is spread through contact with blood. AIDS, hepatitis B, and other blood infections may be undiagnosed. Universal precautions prevent the spread of AIDS and other infections. Therefore, universal precautions are used for *all* residents of nursing facilities.

As a nurse aide, you will not insert needles into the resident's body or obtain blood for laboratory study. However, you may care for residents who have bleeding wounds. Their linens, gowns, pajamas, or clothing could become soiled with blood. Contact with blood may occur when giving oral hygiene to someone with bleeding gums, or a resident can be nicked when being shaved. There may be blood or pathogens in urine, feces, vomitus, respiratory secretions, or vaginal secretions. There are many other situations in which you could have contact with a resident's blood or body fluids.

Universal precautions involve setting up barriers to prevent contact with the resident's blood, body fluids, or body substances. *The Centers for Disease Control recommend the use of universal precautions for all residents.* Your facility will have policies regarding the use of universal precautions, which are described in the box on p. 30.

UNIVERSAL PRECAUTIONS

Gloves are worn when touching blood, body fluids, body substances, and mucous membranes.

Gloves are worn when there are cuts, breaks, or openings in the skin.

Gloves are worn when there is possible contact with urine, feces, vomitus, dressings, wound drainage, soiled linen, or soiled clothing.

Masks, goggles, or face shields are worn when splattering or splashing of blood or body fluids is possible. (This protects your eyes and the mucous membranes of your mouth.)

Gowns or aprons are worn when splashing, splattering, smearing, or soiling from blood or body fluids is possible.

Hands and other body parts must be washed immediately if contaminated with blood or body fluids.

Hands are washed immediately after removing gloves.

Hands are washed after contact with a resident.

Avoid nicks or cuts when shaving residents.

Handle razor blades and other sharp objects carefully to avoid injuring the resident or yourself.

Use resuscitation devices (not mouth-to-mouth) when resuscitation is indicated.

Avoid resident contact when you have open skin wounds or lesions. Discuss the situation with your charge nurse.

SUMMARY

Preventing the spread of infection is the responsibility of every health care worker. You must be conscientious about your work. Your employer and your residents assume that you will practice medical asepsis and universal precautions to prevent the spread of microorganisms and infection. The simple procedure of handwashing before and after resident contact does a lot to reduce the spread of microorganisms.

CHAPTER 3

Safety and Emergency Procedures

Objectives

Identify safety measures that prevent accidents in the home

Describe the safety measures that prevent falls

Identify common safety hazards in health-care facilities

Explain seven reasons why people may be unable to protect themselves

Describe the types of restraints and safety rules for using them

Identify common equipment-related accidents and how they can be prevented

Identify accidents and errors that need to be reported

Describe safety measures related to fire prevention and the use of oxygen

Know what to do if there is a fire and how to use a fire extinguisher

Give examples of natural and man-made disasters

Safety is a basic need. People need to be safe from accidents and dangers. Homes and health-care facilities are thought to be free of dangers and hazards. This is not true. Many accidental injuries occur in the home. Some cause death. Accidents also occur in health-care facilities.

You are responsible for safe practices at home and in everyday activities. When caring for residents you need to practice ordinary safety precautions and the other safety measures presented in this chapter.

THE SAFE ENVIRONMENT

A safe environment is one in which a person has a low risk of becoming ill or injured. The person feels safe and secure both physically and psychologically. There is little risk of developing an infection, falling, being burned or poisoned, or suffering other injuries. The person is comfortable in relation to temperature, noise, and smells. There is enough lighting and room to move about.

SAFETY IN THE HOME

Most accidents in the home can be prevented. Common sense and simple safety measures help eliminate some causes of accidental injuries. Nurse aides employed by home health care agencies should see that measures have been taken to prevent accidents in the home. The nurse should be consulted if safety hazards are present.

Falls

Falls are the most common home accidents, especially among the elderly. Most falls occur in bedrooms and bathrooms. They are usually due to slippery floors, throw rugs, poor lighting, cluttered floors, furniture that is out of place, and slippery bathtubs or showers. The following measures can help prevent falls in the home.

1. Provide good lighting in rooms and hallways.
2. Install hand rails on both sides of stairs and in bathrooms.
3. Use wall-to-wall carpeting or carpeting that is tacked down. Avoid "throw rugs".
4. Use nonskid shoes and slippers.
5. Use nonskid wax on hardwood, tiled, or linoleum floors.
6. Keep floors uncluttered and free of toys and other objects that can trip someone.
7. Keep electric and extension cords out of the way.
8. Avoid rearranging furniture.
9. Have a telephone and lamp at the bedside.
10. Use nonskid bathmats in tubs and showers.

Burns

Burns are a leading cause of death in the United States, especially among the elderly. Common causes of burns are smoking in bed, spilling hot liquids, charcoal grills, fireplaces, stoves, and bath water being too hot. Safety measures to prevent burns in the home include:

1. Turn the handles of pots and pans on stoves so that they do not extend beyond the edge of the stove where people stand and walk.
2. Supervise the smoking of adults who are unable to protect themselves.
3. Prohibit smoking in bed.
4. Test the bath water or shower temperature before entering.

Poisoning

Accidental poisoning is another major cause of death. Poisoning in adults may be accidental from decreased awareness, carelessness, or poor vision when reading labels. Sometimes poisoning is a suicide attempt. Most accidental poisoning can be prevented by:

1. Labeling all medicine containers and household products clearly.
2. Storing poisonous materials properly.
3. Storing poisonous materials in their original containers and not in food containers.
4. Making sure that there is adequate lighting so that labels can be read accurately.

Suffocation

Suffocation is when breathing stops due to a lack of oxygen. Death occurs if the person does not start breathing again. Common causes of suffocation include choking on an object, drowning, inhaling gas or smoke, strangulation, and electrical shock. Safety measures to help prevent suffocation are:

1. Taking small bites of food and chewing food slowly and thoroughly.
2. Having gas odors promptly investigated by a competent repairman.
3. Opening doors and windows if gas odors are noted.
4. Making sure electrical cords and appliances are in good repair.

SAFETY IN THE HEALTH CARE FACILITY

Safety hazards also exist in health-care facilities. The measures that promote safety in the home also apply in health-care facilities. However, additional safety measures are needed in the health-care facility.

Identifying your resident

You will care for several residents while on duty. Each has different treatments, therapies, and activity limitations. Residents must be protected from infections, falls, and accidents related to equipment. Safety also involves giving care to the correct resident. A resident's life and health can be threatened if the wrong care is given.

Residents of nursing facilities receive identification (ID) bracelets when admitted to the facility or have ID pictures placed on Kardex. It is important to check either the ID bracelet or picture before giving care.

You should also call the person by name while checking the ID bracelet or picture. Calling the resident by name is a courtesy that should be given as the person is being touched and before care is given. However, calling the resident by name is not a reliable way to identify the person. Confused, disoriented, drowsy, or hearing-impaired residents may answer to any name.

Preventing falls

Falls are common safety problems in health-care facilities. Residents have problems that can cause falls, such as weakness from illness, a strange environment and new medications.

The safety measures to prevent falls in the home apply to health-care facilities. Side rails, hand rails, and restraints are some safety devices used to prevent falls.

Side rails. Side rails are attached to the sides of hospital beds. They can be raised or lowered, and are locked in place by levers, latches, or buttons. They protect the resident from falling out of bed. Residents can use side rails to move and turn in bed. Side rails can be half the length or the full length of a bed.

Side rails are necessary for residents who are unconscious, sedated with medication, confused, or disoriented. Side rails should be kept up at all times for these residents, except when giving care.

Some residents find the use of side rails embarrassing. They feel that they are being treated like children. Some facilities do not require side rails if the resident signs a statement releasing the facility of responsibility for falls. If a resident objects to side rails, report the concern to the nurse. Residents must be protected physically, but their psychological need for esteem must also be protected.

Hand rails. Hand rails are installed in hallways and bathrooms of nursing facilities. They provide support for residents who are weak or unsteady when walking. They also provide support when sitting down on or getting up from a toilet. Hand rails may be found along bathtubs for use in getting in and out of the tub. Hand rails are always found in stairways.

Other safety measures. You need to practice other safety measures to prevent patients from falling.

1. Keep the resident's bed in the lowest horizontal position, except when giving bedside nursing care. The distance from the bed to floor is reduced if the resident falls or gets out of bed.
2. Have a night-light on in the resident's room.
3. Keep floors free of spills and excess furniture.
4. Have residents wear nonskid shoes or slippers when out of bed rather than soft bedroom slippers.
5. Make sure that crutches, canes, and walkers have nonskid tips which prevent slipping or skidding on floors.
6. Keep the signal or call light within reach at all times. The resident should be taught how to use the light and to call for help whenever help is needed.

7. Lock the wheels of beds, wheelchairs, and stretchers when helping residents get in or out of them.
8. Use caution when turning corners, entering corridor intersections, and going through doors. You could bump into a person coming from the opposite direction, causing an injury.

SOME PEOPLE CANNOT PROTECT THEMSELVES

There are many reasons why some individuals cannot protect themselves and are at greater risk. Age, impaired vision, and impaired hearing are factors that cause persons to be at greater risk, along with disorientation and paralysis. Medication can also cause a variety of side effects on people. You need to be aware of any factors that increase a resident's risk of an accident so that you can provide for their safety.

Restraints (protective devices)

Restraints, also called protective devices, are used to protect residents from harming themselves or others. The resident may be confined to a bed or chair or prevented from moving a body part. Restraints are applied to the chest, waist, elbows, wrists, or ankles. They are made of either linen or leather.

There are certain considerations you must understand about using restraints.

1. *Restraints are used to protect residents, not for the convenience of the staff.* A restraint is used only when it is the best safety precaution for the resident. They should not be used to punish uncooperative residents.
2. *Restraints require a doctor's order.* OBRA and state laws protect individuals from being restrained unnecessarily. Health care facilities also have policies and procedures about using restraints. If a resident needs to be restrained for medical purposes, there must be a written doctor's order. The doctor is usually required by law to give the reason for the restraint. The order and its reason will be on the resident's Kardex. You need to know the laws and policies about using restraints where you work.
3. *Unnecessary restraint of a resident constitutes false imprisonment, which is the unlawful restraint or restriction of a person's freedom of movement.* If you are told to apply a restraint, the need for it should be clearly evident and understood. If not, politely request an explanation.
4. *The restrained resident's basic needs must be met by the nursing team.* The restraint should be tied to the bedframe using a square knot for easy removal (Fig. 3-1). The restraint should be firm, but not tight. Padding may be used to protect skin and bony areas. A tight restraint may interfere with circulation or breathing. Movement of the restrained part should be possible to a limited

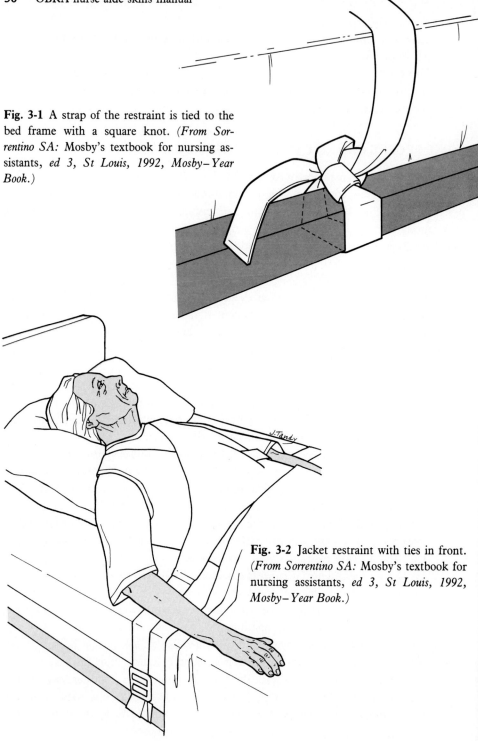

Fig. 3-1 A strap of the restraint is tied to the bed frame with a square knot. (*From Sorrentino SA:* Mosby's textbook for nursing assistants, *ed 3, St Louis, 1992, Mosby–Year Book.*)

Fig. 3-2 Jacket restraint with ties in front. (*From Sorrentino SA:* Mosby's textbook for nursing assistants, *ed 3, St Louis, 1992, Mosby–Year Book.*)

and safe extent. The resident and family should be given an explanation by the nurse about the need and purpose of the restraint. The resident must be checked often (every 15 minutes; skin color and warmth should be reported). Restraints should be removed every 2 hours and skin care given.

5. *Restraints may have to be applied rapidly.* They need to be applied with enough assistance to protect the resident and staff from injury. Residents who are in immediate danger of harming themselves or others need to be restrained quickly. Combative and agitated residents can injure themselves and the staff when the restraints are being applied. Enough staff members are needed to complete the task safely and efficiently.

6. *A resident may become more confused or agitated after being restrained.* Even when confused, residents are aware of restricted body movements. They may try to get out of the restraint, or struggle or pull at the restraint. These behaviors are often misinterpreted as confusion. Confused residents may become more confused because they do not understand what is happening to them. The resident needs repeated explanations and reassurance. Spending time with the resident often has a calming effect.

Reporting and recording. Certain information about restraints must be included in the resident's record. You may be instructed to apply restraints or be assigned to care for a restrained resident. The following must be reported to the nurse.

1. The type of restraint applied.
2. The time of application.
3. The time when the restraint was removed.
4. The type of care given when the restraint was removed.
5. The color and condition of the resident's skin.
6. Whether or not a pulse is felt in the restrained extremity.
7. Resident complaints of pain, numbness, or tingling in the restrained part.

Wrist and ankle restraints. Wrist and ankle restraints are also called hand and foot restraints. They are used to limit the movement of an arm or leg.

Mitt restraints. A resident's hands are placed in mitt restraints. They prevent use of the fingers, but do not prevent hand or wrist movements. The arms can also be immobilized by securing the straps to the bed frame. Mitt restraints are thumbless and prevent the resident from scratching, pulling out tubes, or removing dressings. The resident may be given a hand roll to grasp so that the fingers are kept in a normal position.

Jacket restraints. Jacket restraints are applied to the chest to protect the patient from falling out of a bed or chair. The resident's arms are put through the sleeves so that the vest crosses in front (Fig. 3-2). The vest should *never* cross in the back. The restraint is always applied over a gown, pajamas, or clothes.

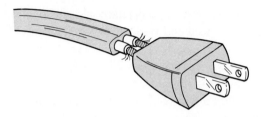

Fig. 3-3 A frayed electric wire. (*From Sorrentino SA:* Mosby's textbook for nursing assistants, *ed 3, St Louis, 1992, Mosby–Year Book.*)

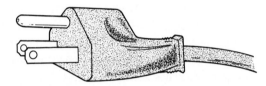

Fig. 3-4 Three pronged plug. (*From Sorrentino SA:* Mosby's textbook for nursing assistants, *ed 3, St Louis, 1992, Mosby–Year Book.*)

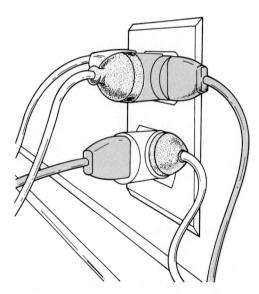

Fig. 3-5 An overloaded electrical outlet. (*From Sorrentino SA:* Mosby's textbook for nursing assistants, *ed 3, St Louis, 1992, Mosby–Year Book.*)

Safety belt or waist restraint. The safety belt or waist restraint is used for the same reasons as the jacket restraint. The belt is applied around the waist and secured to the bed or chair. The belt is applied over clothes, a gown, or pajamas.

Accidents due to equipment

Glass and plastic equipment must be intact and inspected before use. The equipment is checked for cracks, chips, and sharp or rough edges which can cut, stab, or scratch residents. Damaged equipment should not be used or given to residents. Instead, take the item to the nurse, point out the defect, and discard the item as instructed.

Electrical equipment must function properly and be in good repair. Frayed cords (Fig. 3-3) can cause electrical shocks that result in death. Fires may also result. Frayed cords and defective equipment must be repaired by a trained individual.

Three-pronged plugs (Fig. 3-4) should be used on all equipment. Two prongs carry electrical current and the third prong is a ground. A *ground* is protection from a "short" in a defective piece of equipment. Leaking electricity can therefore be conducted to a person, creating shocks and possible death. Be sure to report a piece of equipment that gives you a shock while using it. The item should be sent for repair.

Reporting accidents and errors. Accidents and errors must be reported immediately to your supervisor. This includes accidents involving residents, visitors, or staff. You must report errors in resident care. Such errors include giving a resident a wrong treatment, giving a treatment to the wrong resident, or forgetting to give a treatment. Breakage of items owned by the resident, such as dentures or eye glasses, must be reported. Loss of a resident's money or clothing must also be reported.

When reporting accidents or errors, you need to give the names of those involved, date, time, and location of the accident or error. You also need to provide a complete description of what happened, names of witnesses, and other requested information. Most facilities require written reports about the accident or error. These are called "incident reports."

FIRE SAFETY

Faulty electrical equipment and wiring, overloaded electrical circuits (Fig. 3-5), and smoking are major causes of fire. Fire is a constant danger in homes and health-care facilities. The entire health team is responsible for preventing fires and for acting quickly and responsibly in the event of a fire.

Fire and the use of oxygen

Three things are needed to start and maintain a fire: a spark or flame, a material that will burn, and oxygen. There is a certain amount of oxygen found in the air. However, some residents need more oxygen than is available in the air. Doctors order supplemental oxygen for these residents. Supplemental oxygen is supplied in portable oxygen tanks or through wall outlets. Because supplemental oxygen increases the risk of fires, special safety precautions are practiced where oxygen is being given and stored. They are:

1. "No Smoking" signs are placed on the resident's door and near the bed.
2. Residents and visitors are politely reminded not to smoke in the resident's room.
3. Smoking materials (cigarettes, cigars, and pipes), matches, and lighters belonging to the resident are removed from the room.
4. Electrical equipment is turned off before being unplugged. Sparks occur when electrical appliances are unplugged while still turned on.
5. Wool blankets and synthetic fabrics that cause static electricity are removed from the resident's room.
6. Electrical equipment is removed from the room. This includes electric razors, heating pads, and radios.
7. Materials that ignite easily are removed from the resident's room. These include oil, grease, alcohol, and nail polish remover.

Fire prevention

Fire prevention measures have been described about burns in the home, equipment-related accidents, and the use of oxygen. These and other fire safety measures are summarized as follows.

1. Follow the fire safety precautions related to the use of supplemental oxygen.
2. Smoke only in areas where smoking is allowed.
3. Be sure all ashes and cigar and cigarette butts are out before emptying ashtrays.
4. Provide ashtrays to residents who are allowed to smoke.
5. Empty ashtrays into a metal container partially filled with sand or water. Do not empty ashtrays into plastic containers or wastebaskets lined with paper or plastic bags.
6. Supervise residents who are unable to protect themselves when they smoke. This includes confused, disoriented, and sedated patients.
7. Follow necessary safety practices when using electrical equipment.

What to do if there is a fire

Each health-care facility has policies and procedures explaining what to do if there is a fire. You must know them for your facility. Also know the location of the fire alarms, fire extinguishers, and emergency exits. Fire drills are held in all facilities so that the procedures can be practiced.

The following practices are usually carried out by the health team when there is a fire.

1. Sound the nearest fire alarm.
2. Notify the switchboard operator of the exact location of the fire.
3. Move residents who are in the immediate area of the fire to a safe place.
4. Use a fire extinguisher on a small fire that has not spread to a large area.
5. Turn off any oxygen or electrical equipment being used in the general area of the fire.
6. Close all doors and windows.
7. Clear all regular and emergency exits of equipment.
8. Do not use elevators if there is a fire.

You should be able to use a fire extinguisher. Fire departments often give demonstrations on how to use fire extinguishers to employees of health-care facilities. These demonstrations are given once or twice a year. Some facilities require all employees to be able to use a fire extinguisher.

There are different extinguishers for different kinds of fires: oil and grease fires, electrical fires, and paper and wood fires. A general procedure for using a fire extinguisher follows.

1. Pull the fire alarm.
2. Get the nearest fire extinguisher.
3. Carry the extinguisher so it is upright.
4. Take the extinguisher to the fire.
5. Remove the safety pin.
6. Push the top handle down.
7. Direct the hose at the base of the fire.

DISASTERS

A *disaster* is a sudden, catastrophic event. Many people are injured or killed and property is destroyed. Disasters may be natural, such as tornados, hurricanes, blizzards, earthquakes, volcanic eruptions, and floods. Man-made disasters include automobile, bus, train, and airplane accidents; fires; nuclear power plant accidents; riots; explosions; and wars.

Local communities and health-care facilities have disaster plans. You should be familiar with the disaster plan where you work and the disaster plan of the community where you live and work.

SUMMARY

Most accidents can be prevented. Knowing the common safety hazards and accidents, knowing who needs protection, and common sense are all necessary to promote safety. The elderly and individuals who are disoriented, paralyzed, or who have vision and hearing losses are more likely to have accidents than healthy people.

Illness, medications, strange surroundings, and special equipment also increase the risk of accidental injury. As a nurse aide, you need to practice safety precautions, use side rails, and encourage residents to use hand rails.

The importance of identifying residents before giving care must be emphasized. The resident's life and health can be seriously threatened if the wrong care is given or if care is omitted.

If restraints are ordered, they must be used only to protect the resident or to prevent the resident from harming others. The resident must be checked often to make sure that breathing and circulation are normal. Remember that the restrained resident depends on others for meeting basic needs. Also remember that you can be charged with false imprisonment if a resident is restrained unnecessarily.

Fire is a safety hazard. Safety precautions applied to smoking and use of electrical equipment help prevent fires. Extra precautions are needed when supplemental oxygen is being used. Be sure you know where fire alarms, fire extinguishers, and emergency exits are located. Also be sure you know what to do if there is a fire. Safety is everyone's concern.

CHAPTER 4

Promoting Residents' Adjustment, Independence, and Rights

Objectives

Identify the developmental tasks of late adulthood (elderly)

Identify physical and psychosocial losses residents experience that decrease their independence

Describe losses residents experience when they enter a nursing facility

Identify ways in which nurse aides can assist a resident to cope with losses

The number of people over 65 years of age is increasing every day. Individuals are living longer and are healthier. Most people can expect to live into their 70s. A hundred years ago most people died in their 50s. Many individuals in their 70s and 80s today continue to live healthy and happy lives in their homes.

Physical, psychological, and social changes occur during later adulthood. People in this stage of development are often referred to as the elderly.

The developmental tasks of the elderly are:

1. Adjusting to decreased physical strength and loss of health.
2. Adjusting to retirement and reduced income.
3. Coping with the death of a husband or wife.
4. Developing new friends and relationships.
5. Preparing for one's death.

PSYCHOLOGICAL AND SOCIAL EFFECTS OF AGING

Physical, psychological, and social changes occur as a person gets older. Graying hair, wrinkles, and slow movements are physical reminders of growing old. Retirement from a job and the death of a spouse, relatives, and friends are social reminders. Society values youth and beauty. This emphasis can make growing old an emotionally painful process.

Retirement

People traditionally retire at the age of 65. Some retire earlier. Others continue to work until the age of 70 or beyond. Retirement is viewed as a reward for a lifetime of work. The individual has earned the right not to work and can now relax and enjoy life. Travel, leisure, and doing whatever one wants are the "benefits" of retirement. Many people are able to enjoy retirement, while others are not so fortunate. Some must retire because of chronic disease or disability. Poor health and medical expenses can make the enjoyment of retirement very difficult.

Working has social and psychological effects. Work helps meet the basic needs of love, belonging, and self-esteem. Personal satisfaction and usefulness result from working. Friendships develop and day-to-day events are shared with co-workers. Leisure activities, recreation, and companionship often involve co-workers. Some individuals rely upon work for psychological and social fulfillment. Retirement can be difficult for them. Some retired people have part-time jobs or do volunteer work. Such activities promote usefulness and well-being.

Retirement usually means reduced income. The monthly social security check may be the only source of income. However, retirement and aging do not always mean fewer expenses. There may still be rent or mortgage payments. Food, clothing, gas and electricity, water bills, and taxes are other expenses. Car expenses, home repairs, medicine, and health care are additional costs. For many people, retirement causes severe financial problems. Other people are able to plan for retirement through savings, investments, retirement plans, and insurance coverage.

Social relationships

Social relationships change throughout life. Children have grown and left home and may have families of their own. Many live far away from their elderly parents. Elderly friends and relatives may have moved away, died, or are disabled. Loneliness may be experienced. Separation from children and the lack of companionship with people their own age are common causes of loneliness in the elderly.

Many elderly people are able to adjust to these changes. Hobbies, church, community activities, and new friends help prevent loneliness. Being a grandparent can be a source of great love and enjoyment. Being included in family activities helps prevent loneliness, and it also allows the elderly person to feel useful and wanted.

Some elderly individuals speak and understand only a foreign language. This may cause social problems.

Another social change experienced by some elderly people is being cared for by their children. In this situation parents and children change roles. Instead of the parent caring for the child, the child cares for the parent. This role change and dependency on a child can make the elderly person feel more secure. However, others feel unwanted, in the way of others, and useless. Some feel a loss of dignity or self-respect.

Death of a spouse

As a husband and wife grow older, the chances increase that one of them will die. In general, women live longer than men. Therefore, becoming a widow will be a reality for many women.

A person may try to psychologically prepare for the death of their spouse. When death does occur however, the loss is devastating. No amount of preparation is enough for the emptiness and changes that result. The individual loses more than a husband or wife. A friend, lover, and companion are also lost. The grief felt by the surviving spouse may be very great. Serious physical and mental problems can result. The surviving spouse may lose the will to live or attempt suicide.

PHYSICAL EFFECTS OF AGING

Certain physical changes are a normal part of the aging process and occur in all individuals (Table 2). The rate and degree of change vary with each person. Many changes effect personality and mental functioning. Memory is often shorter and forgetfulness increases. The ability to respond is slower. Confusion, dizziness, and fatigue may also occur. Elderly people often remember events in the distant past better than those in the recent past. Many elderly people keep mentally active and involved in current events. They usually show fewer personality and mental changes.

Less sleep is needed by the elderly. However, loss of energy and decreased blood flow cause fatigue. Usually the elderly rest or nap during the day, then go to bed early and get up early.

NURSING FACILITIES

Nursing facilities are alternatives for the elderly who can no longer care for themselves. These are commonly called nursing homes. Nursing facilities offer different levels of care. Some merely provide room, board, food, and laundry services. Others provide nursing, rehabilitation, dietary, recreational, social, and religious services.

Nursing facilities may be privately owned or operated by the government. In either case, state and federal agencies monitor the care given. State and federal standards required by law must be followed. Periodic inspections, either scheduled or unannounced are held.

Some individuals remain in nursing facilities for the rest of their lives. Others stay until they are able to return to their homes. The nursing facility is the person's

Table 2 Physical changes during the aging process

System	Changes
Musculoskeletal	Muscle atrophy Decreasing strength Bones become brittle and can break easily Joints become stiff and painful Gradual loss of height Decreased mobility
Cardiovascular	Heart pumps with less force Arteries narrow and are less elastic Less blood flows through narrowed arteries
Respiratory	Respiratory muscles weaken Lung tissue becomes less elastic
Urinary	Kidney function decreases Poisonous substances can build up in the blood Urine becomes concentrated Urinary incontinence may occur
Gastrointestinal	Decreased saliva production Difficulty in swallowing Decreased appetite Decreased secretion of digestive juices Fried and fatty foods are difficult to digest Loss of teeth Decreased peristalsis causing flatulence and constipation

Table 2 Physical changes during the aging process—cont'd

System	Changes
Integumentary	Skin becomes less elastic Fatty tissue layer of the skin is lost Folds, lines, and wrinkles appear Dry skin develops Increased sensitivity to cold Nails become thick and tough Whitening or graying hair Loss or thinning of hair
Nervous	Vision and hearing decrease Decreased sense of taste and smell Reduced sense of touch and sensitivity to pain Reduced blood flow to the brain Progressive loss of brain cells Shorter memory Forgetfulness Slowed ability to respond Confusion Dizziness
Reproductive	Changes in reproductive organs Decreased hormone production (estrogen, testosterone) Decreased frequency of sexual activity Menopause (female)

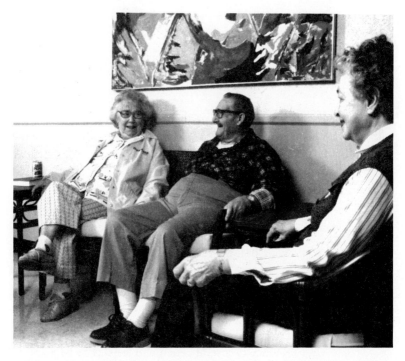

Fig. 4-1 The atmosphere of a long-term care facility is similar to a home. *(From Sorrentino SA:* Mosby's textbook for nursing assistants, *ed 3, St Louis, 1992, Mosby–Year Book.)*

temporary or permanent home. The surroundings are made as home-like as possible (Fig. 4-1). The individual is referred to as a resident.

A resident in the nursing facility feels a great sense of loss. This may include a loss of self-identity, loss of personal belongings and home, loss of independence, and loss of personal choice. The health care team, including the nurse aide, can assist the resident in coping with these changes. The nurse aide can promote privacy, personal choices, and socialization (see Fig. 4-1). The nurse aide should also encourage the resident's participation in activities of daily living (ADL) and in the facility's activities.

SUMMARY

Aging is a normal process. The elderly must adjust to the physical changes that occur, such as graying of hair, loss of physical strength, and loss of health. Retirement, a change of financial situation, and loss of a spouse or friends can cause loneliness and isolation.

Many people fear the possibility of living in a nursing facility. The nurse aide can help a resident cope with losses and meet their basic needs.

CHAPTER 5

Respecting Residents' Rights

Objectives

Identify basic human rights
Discuss ways to protect residents' rights
Define abuse of the elderly and understand the nurse aide's role in reporting abuse

RESIDENT RIGHTS

Residents of nursing facilities have certain rights under federal and state laws. Residents have rights as citizens of the United States. They also have rights relating to their everyday lives and care in a nursing facility. Nursing facilities must protect and promote resident rights. Residents must be able to exercise their rights without interference from the facility. Some residents are incompetent (not able) and cannot exercise their rights. Legal guardians exercise rights for them.

Nursing facilities must inform residents of their rights. They must be informed orally and in writing. Such information is given before or upon admission to the facility. It must be given in the language used and understood by the resident.

Privacy and confidentiality

All residents have a right to privacy and confidentiality. OBRA provides for privacy and confidentiality.

Residents have the right to personal privacy. The resident's body must not be exposed unnecessarily. Only those workers directly involved in care, treatments, or examinations should be present. A resident also has the right to use the bathroom in private. Privacy should also be maintained for personal care activities.

Residents also have the right to visit with others in privacy. They have the right to visit in an area where they cannot be seen or heard by others. The facility must try to provide private space when it is requested. Offices, chapels, dining rooms, meeting rooms, and conference rooms can be used if available.

The right to visit in privacy also involves telephone conversations. Residents also have the right to send and receive mail without interference by others. Letters sent and received by the resident must not be opened by others without the resident's permission.

Information about the resident's care, treatment, and condition must be kept confidential. Medical and financial records are also confidential. The resident must give consent for them to be released to other facilities or individuals. However, consent is not needed for the release of medical records when the resident is being transferred to another facility. Records can also be released without the resident's consent when they are required by law or for insurance purposes.

Providing for privacy and keeping medical and personal information confidential show respect for the individual. They also protect the person's dignity.

Personal choice

OBRA requires that residents be free to choose their physicians. They also have the right to participate in planning their care and treatment. This means that residents have the right to choose activities, schedules, and care based on their personal preferences. For example, residents have the right to choose when to get up and go to bed, what to wear, how to spend their time, and what to eat. They can also choose companions and visitors inside and outside of the nursing facility.

Personal choice is important for quality of life, dignity, and self-respect. You will be reminded to allow the person's preferences whenever it is safely possible.

Disputes and grievances

Residents have the right to voice concerns, questions, and complaints about treatment or care. The dispute or grievance may involve another resident. It may be about treatment or care that was not given. The facility must promptly try to correct the situation. The resident must not be punished in any way for voicing the dispute or grievance.

Participation in resident and family groups

Residents have the right to participate in resident and family groups. This means that residents have the right to form groups. A resident's family has the right to meet with the families of other residents. These groups can discuss concerns and offer suggestions to improve the quality of life in the facility. They can also plan activities for residents and families. The groups can serve to provide support and reassurance for group members. Residents also have the right to participate in social, religious, and community activities. They have the right to assistance in getting to and from activities of their choice.

Care and security of personal possessions

Residents have the right to keep and use personal possessions. Available space and the health and safety of other residents can affect the type and amount of personal possessions allowed. A person's property must be treated with care and respect. Though the items may not have value to you, they are important to the resident. They also relate to personal choice, dignity, and quality of life.

The facility must take reasonable measures to protect the individual's property. Items should be labeled with the resident's name. The facility must investigate reports of lost, stolen, or damaged items. Police assistance is sometimes necessary. The resident and family will probably be advised not to keep jewelry and other expensive items in the facility.

You must protect yourself and the facility from being accused of stealing a resident's property. Do not go through a resident's closet, drawers, purse, or other space without the person's knowledge and consent. Have another worker with you and the resident or legal guardian present if it is necessary to inspect closets and drawers. The worker serves as a witness to your activities.

Freedom from abuse, mistreatment, and neglect

OBRA states that residents have the right to be free from verbal, sexual, physical, or mental abuse.

Residents also have the right to be free from involuntary seclusion. Involuntary seclusion is separating the resident from others against his or her will. It can also mean keeping the person away from his or her room without consent, or being confined to a certain area. If the person is incompetent, involuntary seclusion occurs against the legal guardian's consent.

No one can abuse, neglect, or mistreat the resident. This includes facility staff, volunteers, staff from other agencies or groups, other residents, family, visitors, and legal guardians. Nursing facilities must have policies and procedures for investigating suspected or reported cases of resident abuse. Also, nursing facilities cannot hire someone who has been convicted of abusing, neglecting, or mistreating other individuals.

Freedom from restraints

Residents have the right not to have body movements restricted. Body movements can be restricted by using restraints or certain drugs. Some drugs restrain the person because they affect mood, behavior, and mental functioning. Sometimes residents need to be restrained to protect them from harming themselves or others. A physician's order is necessary for restraints to be used. Restraints cannot be used for the convenience of the staff.

ABUSE OF THE ELDERLY

Abuse of the elderly has become more evident in today's society. The abuser is usually a family member or a person caring for the elderly individual. There are different forms of abuse. In some cases the elderly person may be intentionally harmed.

1. *Physical abuse* involves hitting, slapping, kicking, pinching, and beating. Physical injury and pain may result. Another form of physical abuse is not providing needed medical services or treatment.
2. *Verbal abuse* is the use of spoken or written words that speak ill of, sneer at, criticize, or condemn the resident. OBRA guidelines also include unkind gestures as verbal abuse.
3. *Involuntary seclusion* is confining the person to a specific area. Elderly people have been locked in closets, basements, attics, and other spaces.
4. *Financial abuse* is when the elderly person's money is used by another person.
5. *Mental abuse* relates to humiliation and threats of being punished or not being given such things as food, clothing, care, a home, or a place to sleep.
6. *Sexual abuse* is when the person is harassed about sex or is attacked sexually. The person may be forced to perform sexual acts out of fear of punishment or physical harm.

Abused elderly are found in homes, hospitals, or nursing facilities. Often the abuse is unrecognized. The following are signs of elderly abuse. The abused person may show only some of them.

1. Living conditions are unsafe, unclean, or inadequate.
2. Personal hygiene is lacking. The individual is unclean and clothes are dirty.
3. Weight loss has occurred. There are signs of poor nutrition and inadequate fluid intake.
4. There are frequent injuries. The circumstances behind the injuries are strange or seem unlikely.
5. Old and new bruises are seen.
6. The person seems very quiet or withdrawn.
7. The person seems fearful, anxious, or agitated.
8. The individual does not seem to want to talk or answer questions.
9. The person is restrained or locked in a certain area for long periods of time. Toilet facilities, food, water, and other necessary items cannot be reached.
10. Private conversations are not allowed. The caregiver is present during all conversations.
11. The person seems too anxious to please the caregiver.
12. Medications are not taken properly. Medications are not purchased, or too much or too little medication is taken.
13. Visits to the emergency room may be frequent.
14. The person may go from one doctor to another, or the person does not have a doctor.

OBRA and state laws require that elderly abuse be reported. If abuse is suspected, it must be reported. Where and how to report suspected abuse varies in each state. If you do report suspected abuse, you need to give as much information as possible. The reporting agency will take action based on the information given. They act immediately if there is a life-threatening situation. Sometimes the help of police or the courts is necessary.

Helping the abused elderly is not always easy or possible. The abuse may never be reported or recognized, or the investigating agency may be unable to gain access to the person. Sometimes the elderly are abused by their children, and the victim may want to protect their child. Some victims are embarrassed or feel that the abuse is deserved. A victim may be afraid of what will happen. He or she may feel that the present situation is better than no care at all. Some people feel they will not be believed if they report the abuse themselves.

Elderly abuse is unfortunate. You may suspect that a person is being abused. If so, discuss the situation and your observations with your supervisor. Give the nurse as much information as possible. The nurse will then contact the appropriate members of the health team. The agency that investigates elderly abuse in your community will also be contacted.

SUMMARY

Basic human rights of residents in a nursing facility are to be respected and protected by all health-care workers. Nursing facilities inform residents of their rights upon admission. The rights include privacy; confidentiality; the right of personal choice; the right to voice concerns, questions, and complaints; and the right to participate in group activities. Residents also have the right to be free from abuse, mistreatment, or neglect, and restraint. OBRA requires reporting of elderly abuse. It's important for health-care workers to be aware of resident rights and work to protect them.

CHAPTER 6

Vital Signs

Objectives

Explain why vital signs are measured and factors that can affect vital signs

Identify the normal ranges of oral, rectal, and axillary body temperatures

Know when to take oral, rectal, and axillary temperatures

Identify the sites for taking a pulse and know the normal pulse ranges of different age groups

Describe normal respirations

Know the normal range for adult blood pressure

Describe the difference between mercury and aneroid sphygmomanometers

Describe the practices that you should follow when measuring blood pressure

Vital signs reflect the function of three body processes essential for life: regulation of body temperature, breathing, and heart function. The four *vital signs* of body function are temperature, pulse, respirations, and blood pressure.

Nurse aides often measure vital signs. Accuracy is absolutely essential. You must be accurate in measuring, reporting, and recording vital signs.

MEASURING AND REPORTING VITAL SIGNS

Vital signs are measured to detect changes in normal body function. They are also used to determine a person's response to treatment. Life-threatening situations can also be recognized. Normal temperature, pulse, and respirations (TPR) and blood pressure (BP) will vary within certain limits during any 24-hour period. Many things affect vital signs. They include sleep, activity, eating, weather, noise, exercise, medications, fear, anxiety, and illness.

Vital signs are measured when a person is admitted to a health care facility. Hospital patients have vital signs measured several times a day. The doctor or nurse compares each measurement with previous ones. Residents of nursing facilities do not have their vital signs measured as often. The nurse will tell you when to obtain vital signs. Unless otherwise ordered, vital signs are taken with the person lying or sitting. The person should be at rest when vital signs are measured.

Vital signs reflect even minor changes in a person's condition. They must be measured accurately. If you are unsure of your measurements, promptly ask the nurse to take them again. Vital signs must also be accurately reported and recorded. Any vital sign that is changed from a previous measurement must be reported to the nurse immediately. Vital signs that are above or below the normal range must also be reported immediately.

Many facilities have a "temp board" or a "TPR book." These are divided into columns. The names of individuals are written down the left side of the page. Times of day (such as 8:00 AM, 12:00 PM, 4:00 PM, 8:00 PM) are at the top of the other columns. You will record vital signs in the correct spaces. In some facilities, changed or abnormal vital signs are circled in red. Besides recording them, tell the nurse about changed or abnormal vital signs right away.

BODY TEMPERATURE

Body temperature is the amount of heat in the body. It is a balance between the amount of heat produced and lost by the body. Heat is produced as food is used for energy. It is lost through the skin, by breathing, and by passing urine and feces. A person's body temperature normally remains fairly stable. However, it is slightly lower in the morning and higher in the afternoon and evening. Factors affecting body temperature include age, weather, exercise, pregnancy, menstrual cycles, emotions, and illness.

Normal body temperature

The Fahreheit (F) and Centigrade or Celsius (C) scales are used to measure temperature. Common sites for measuring body temperature are the mouth, rectum, and axilla (underarms). Normal body temperature is 98.6° F (37° C) when measured orally. The normal rectal temperature is 1° higher, or 99.6° F (37.5° C). Normal body temperature ranges for adults are:

Oral: 97.6° to 99.6° F (36.5° to 37.5° C)
Rectal: 98.6° to 100.6° F (37.0° to 38.1° C)
Axillary: 96.6° to 98.6° F (36.0° to 37.0° C)

Types of thermometers

A thermometer is used to measure temperature. The glass thermometer is familiar to most people. There are other kinds of thermometers for measuring body temperature.

Glass thermometers. The glass thermometer (clinical thermometer) is a hollow glass tube with a bulb at one end containing mercury. The mercury rises in the tube when heated by the body. The mercury moves down the tube when cooled.

There are three types of glass thermometers. Each has a different bulb or tip (Fig. 6-1). Long- or slender-tip thermometers are used for oral and axillary temperatures. So are thermometers with stubby- and pear-shaped tips. Rectal thermometers have stubby tips which are color-coded in red. Glass thermometers are available in Fahrenheit and Centigrade scales. Some have both scales.

How to read a glass thermometer. Fahrenheit thermometers have long and short lines. Every other line is marked in an even numbered degree from 94° to 108° F. The short line indicates 0.2 (two-tenths) of a degree (Fig. 6-2). Centigrade thermometers also have long and short lines. Each long line represents one degree, from 34° to 42° C. Each short line represents 0.1 (one-tenth) of a degree (Fig. 6-2). Table 3 shows equivalent values for Fahrenheit and Centigrade scales.

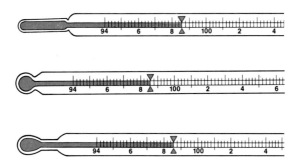

Fig. 6-1 Types of glass thermometers. (*From Sorrentino SA:* Mosby's textbook for nursing assistants, *ed 3, St Louis, 1992, Mosby–Year Book.*)

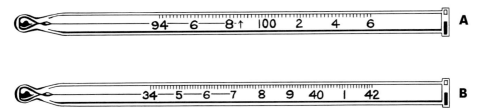

Fig. 6-2 A, Fahrenheit thermometer. **B,** Centigrade thermometer. (*From Sorrentino SA:* Mosby's textbook for nursing assistants, *ed 3, St Louis, 1992, Mosby–Year Book.*)

Table 3 Fahrenheit and Centigrade equivalents

Fahrenheit	Centigrade
95.0	35.0
95.9	35.5
96.8	36.0
97.7	36.5
98.6	37.0
99.5	37.5
100.4	38.0
101.3	38.5
102.2	39.0
103.1	39.5
104.0	40.0
104.9	40.5
105.8	41.0
106.7	41.5
107.6	42.0
108.5	42.5
109.4	43.0
110.3	43.5

Using a glass thermometer. The thermometer is inserted into the mouth, rectum, or axilla. Each of these areas has many microorganisms. A separate thermometer is used for each resident to prevent the spread of microbes and infection. Thermometers are disinfected after use. They are often stored in a disinfectant solution. Before being used again a thermometer is rinsed under cold, running water and wiped with a tissue to remove the disinfectant.

Methods for cleaning thermometers vary among facilities. The thermometer is usually first wiped with a tissue to remove mucus or feces. Then it is washed in cold, soapy water. Hot water is not used. It causes the mercury to expand so much

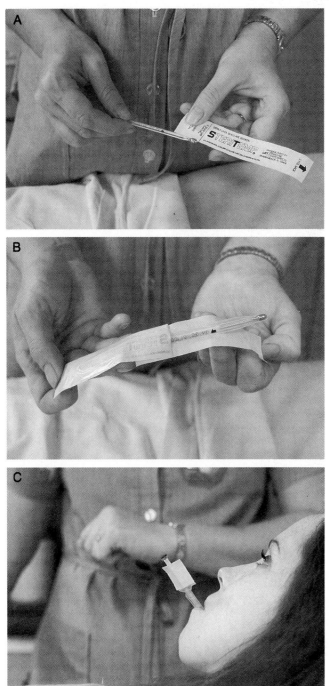

Fig. 6-3 A-C, Glass thermometer and plastic cover. *(From Sorrentino SA:* Mosby's textbook for nursing assistants, *ed 3, St Louis, 1992, Mosby–Year Book.)*

that the thermometer could break. After cleaning, thermometers are rinsed under cold, running water. They are stored in a case or a container filled with disinfectant solution.

Many facilities use plastic covers for thermometers (Fig. 6-3). A cover is used once and then discarded. The thermometer is inserted into a cover and the temperature is taken. The cover is removed to read the thermometer. The thermometer is then inserted into a clean cover and is ready for use. Disinfection and cleaning are not necessary because the thermometer never touches the patient.

Before taking a temperature, the thermometer is shaken down to move the mercury into the bulb. It is checked for breaks or chips which could cause injury to a resident.

HOW TO READ A GLASS THERMOMETER

1. Make sure you have good lighting.
2. Hold the thermometer at the stem with your thumb and fingertips (Fig. 6-4).
3. Bring the thermometer to eye level (Fig. 6-5).
4. Rotate the thermometer until you can see both the numbers and the long and short lines.
5. Note that each long line measures 1 degree and each small line measures 0.1 degrees on a Centigrade thermometer. Each small line on a Fahrenheit thermometer represents 0.2 degrees.
6. Turn the thermometer back and forth slowly until the silver (or red) mercury line is seen.
7. Read the thermometer to the nearest degree (long line). Read the nearest tenth of a degree (short line)—an even number if a Fahrenheit thermometer.
8. Record the resident's name and temperature.

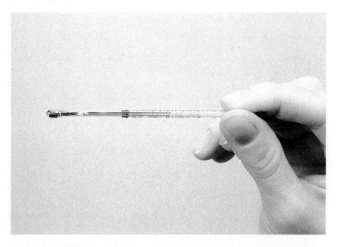

Fig. 6-4 Thermometer is held at the stem with thumb and fingertips. (*From Sorrentino SA: Mosby's textbook for nursing assistants, ed 3, St Louis, 1992, Mosby–Year Book.*)

HOW TO USE A GLASS THERMOMETER

1. Identify yourself to the resident
2. Collect the following equipment:
   - Thermometer
   - Tissues
3. Wash your hands.
4. Hold the thermometer at the stem.
5. Rinse the thermometer under cold running water if it was soaking in a disinfectant. Dry it with tissues from the stem to the bulb end.
6. Shake down the thermometer. The mercury must be below the lines and numbers.
   - Hold the thermometer at the stem.
   - Stand away from walls, tables, or other hard surfaces to avoid breaking the thermometer.
   - Flex and snap your wrist until the mercury is shaken down (Fig. 6-6).
7. Take the resident's temperature.
8. Shake down the thermometer after use.
9. Wipe the thermometer with tissues. Clean it if plastic covers are not used.
10. Place the thermometer in a disinfectant solution or in a plastic cover.

Electronic thermometers. Electronic thermometers are portable and battery operated (Fig. 6-7). They measure a person's temperature in 2 to 60 seconds. The temperature is displayed on the front of the instrument. The hand-held unit is kept in a battery charger when not in use.

Oral and rectal probes are supplied with electronic thermometers. A disposable cover or sheath covers the probes. Disposable probe covers are used only once and then discarded.

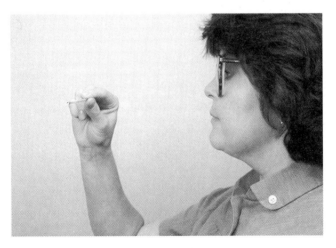

Fig. 6-5 Thermometer is read at eye level. (*From Sorrentino SA:* Mosby's textbook for nursing assistants, *ed 3, St Louis, 1992, Mosby–Year Book.*)

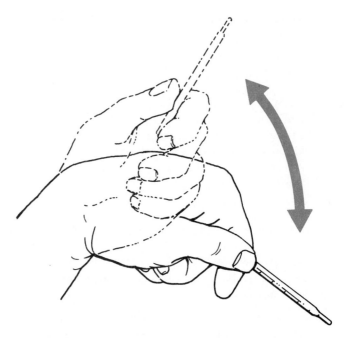

Fig. 6-6 The wrist is snapped to shake down the thermometer. (*From Sorrentino SA:* Mosby's textbook for nursing assistants, *ed 3, St Louis, 1992, Mosby–Year Book.*)

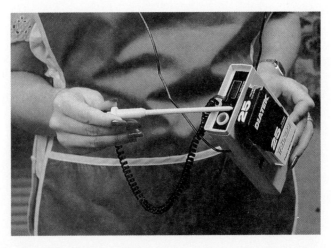

Fig. 6-7 An electronic thermometer. (*From Sorrentino SA:* Mosby's textbook for nursing assistants, *ed 3, St Louis, 1992, Mosby–Year Book.*)

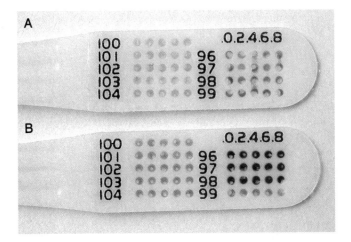

Fig. 6-8 A, Disposable oral thermometer with chemical dots. **B,** The dots change color after the temperature has been taken. *(From Sorrentino SA:* Mosby's textbook for nursing assistants, *ed 3, St Louis, 1992, Mosby–Year Book.)*

Electronic thermometers are expensive. However, they have several advantages. Disposable probe covers reduce the possibility of spreading infection. The temperature display is easily read and the temperature is measured rapidly.

Disposable oral thermometers. Disposable oral thermometers (Fig. 6-8) have small chemical dots. The dots change color when heated by the body. Each dot must be heated to a certain temperature before it changes color. These thermometers are used only once. They measure the temperature in about 45 seconds.

Taking oral temperatures

Oral temperatures are usually taken on older children and adults. Hot and cold foods or fluids, smoking, and chewing gum cause inaccurate measurements. If the resident has done any of these activities, wait 15 minutes before taking an oral temperature. The glass thermometer needs to remain in place 2 to 3 minutes for an accurate measurement. The electronic thermometer probe needs to remain in place until a tone is heard or a flashing light is noted. The disposable thermometer remains in place 45 seconds.

Temperatures should not be taken orally if the resident:

1. Is unconscious
2. Is receiving oxygen
3. Breathes through the mouth
4. Has a sore mouth

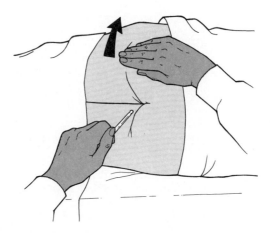

Fig. 6-9 The rectal temperature is taken with the resident in Sim's position. *(From Sorrentino SA: Mosby's textbook for nursing assistants, ed 3, St Louis, 1992, Mosby–Year Book.)*

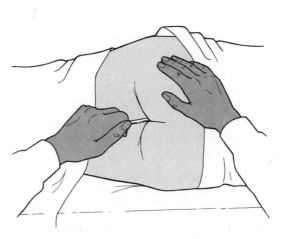

Fig. 6-10 The rectal thermometer is held in place during the measurement. *(From Sorrentino SA: Mosby's textbook for nursing assistants, ed 3, St Louis, 1992, Mosby–Year Book.)*

Taking rectal temperature

The rectal temperature is the most accurate and reliable measurement of body temperature. This route is used when oral temperatures cannot be taken. Rectal temperatures are not taken if the resident has diarrhea, a rectal disorder or injury, heart disease, or after rectal surgery. The resident should be positioned in the Sim's position.

The rectal thermometer is lubricated for easy insertion and to prevent tissue injury. The thermometer is held in place about one-half inch into the rectum, so that it is not broken or lost into the rectum. A glass thermometer must remain in the rectum for 3 minutes for an accurate measurement. The electronic thermometer must remain in place until a tone is heard or a light flashes. Always record an "R" with the measurement (Figs. 6-9 and 6-10).

Taking axillary temperatures

Axillary temperatures are less reliable than oral or rectal temperatures. They are used when the temperature cannot be measured orally or rectally. This site should not be used right after the axilla has been bathed. The axilla should be dry for the measurement. The thermometer must be held in place to maintain proper the position. A glass thermometer is held in place for 9 to 10 minutes for a reliable measurement (Fig. 6-11). An electronic thermometer needs to remain in place until a tone is heard or a light flashes.

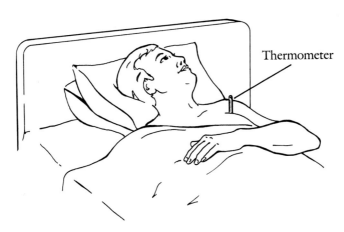

Thermometer

Fig. 6-11 A thermometer is held in place in the axilla by bringing the resident's arm over the chest. (*From Sorrentino SA:* Mosby's textbook for nursing assistants, *ed 3, St Louis, 1992, Mosby–Year Book.*)

PULSE

The *pulse* is felt at an artery as a wave of blood passes through the artery. A pulse can be felt every time the heart beats.

Pulse rate

The *pulse rate* is the number of heartbeats or pulses felt in 1 minute. The pulse rate is influenced by many factors. They include elevated body temperature (fever), exercise, fear, anger, anxiety, excitement, heat, position, and pain. These and other factors cause the heart to beat faster. Some medications also increase the pulse rate. Other drugs slow down the pulse rate.

The adult pulse rate is between 60 and 100 beats per minute. A rate less than 60 or greater than 100 is abnormal. Abnormal rates are reported to the nurse immediately.

Rhythm and force of the pulse

When taking a pulse attention is given to its rhythm and force. The rhythm should be regular. That is, a pulse should be felt in a pattern. The same time interval should occur between beats. An irregular pulse occurs when the beats are unevenly spaced or beats are skipped. The force of the pulse relates to its strength. A forceful pulse is easy to feel and is described as strong, full, or bounding. Pulses that are hard to feel are described as weak, thready, or feeble.

Electronic blood pressure equipment also counts pulses. The pulse rate is displayed along with the blood pressure. However, no information is given about the rhythm and force of the pulse. If electronic blood pressure equipment is used, you still need to feel the pulse to determine rhythm and force.

Using a stethoscope

A *stethoscope* is an instrument used to listen to the sounds produced by the heart, lungs, and other body organs. The stethoscope amplifies the sounds so they can be heard easily. The parts of a stethoscope are shown in Fig. 6-12. The earpieces should fit snugly to block out external noises. However, they should not cause ear pain or discomfort.

Stethoscopes are expensive and are shared by doctors and the nursing team. Care must be taken when using stethoscopes since they will be in contact with many residents and workers. The earpieces and diaphragm are cleaned before and after use. Cleaning prevents the spread of microorganisms. To use a stethoscope for taking a pulse, place the earpieces in the ears and place the diaphragm over the artery.

Sites for taking a pulse

The pulse can be taken at a number of sites (Fig. 6-13) where it is easy to feel. At these sites the arteries are close to the body's surface and lie over a bone. The

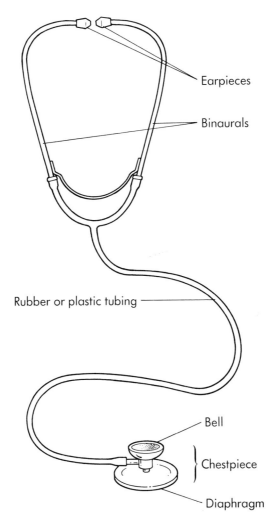

Fig. 6-12 Parts of a stethoscope. *(From Sorrentino SA:* Mosby's textbook for nursing assistants, *ed 3, St Louis, 1992, Mosby–Year Book.)*

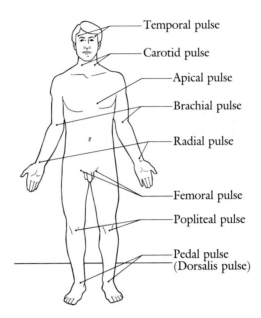

Fig. 6-13 Pulse sites. *(From Sorrentino SA:* Mosby's textbook for nursing assistants, *ed 3, St Louis, 1992, Mosby–Year Book.)*

radial site is used most often because it is easily accessible. The radial pulse can be taken without disturbing or exposing the resident.

Temporal, carotid, brachial, radial, femoral, popliteal, and dorsalis pedis (pedal) arteries are found on both sides of the body. The apical pulse is felt over the apex of the heart. It is taken with a stethoscope.

Taking a radial pulse. The radial pulse is used for routine vital signs. The pulse is felt by placing the first three fingers of one hand against the radial artery. The radial artery is on the thumb side of the wrist (Fig. 6-14). Do not use your thumb to take a pulse; the thumb has a pulse of its own. The pulse in your thumb could be mistaken for the resident's pulse. The pulse is counted for 30 seconds. The number is multiplied by 2 to obtain the number of beats per minute. If the pulse is irregular, it is counted for 1 full minute.

Taking an apical pulse. The apical pulse is taken with a stethoscope. Apical pulses are taken on adults who have heart diseases or who are taking medications that affect the heart. The apical pulse is on the left side of the chest slightly below the nipple (Fig. 6-15). The apical pulse is counted for 1 full minute.

The heartbeat normally sounds like a "lub-dub." Each "lub-dub" is counted as one beat. Do not count the "lub" as one beat and the "dub" as another.

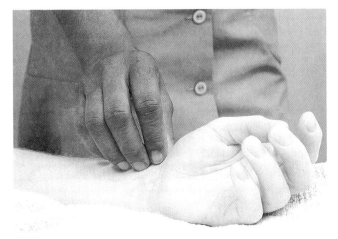

Fig. 6-14 The middle three fingers are used to locate the radial pulse on the thumb side of the wrist. *(From Sorrentino SA:* Mosby's textbook for nursing assistants, *ed 3, St Louis, 1992, Mosby–Year Book.)*

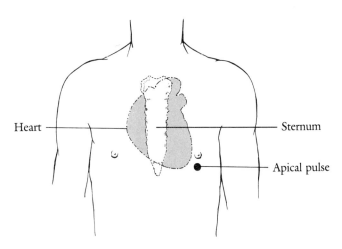

Fig. 6-15 The apical pulse is located 2 to 3 inches to the left of the sternum (breast bone) and below the left nipple. *(From Sorrentino SA:* Mosby's textbook for nursing assistants, *ed 3, St Louis, 1992, Mosby–Year Book.)*

Taking an apical-radial pulse. The apical and radial pulse rates should be equal. Sometimes heart contractions are not strong enough to create pulses in the radial artery. This may occur in people with heart disease. The radial pulse may be less than the apical pulse. To see if there is a difference between the apical and radial rates, the pulses are taken at the same time by two workers. This is called an *apical-radial pulse*. The *pulse deficit* is the difference between the apical and radial pulse rates. To obtain the pulse deficit, subtract the radial rate from the apical rate. The apical pulse is never less than the radial pulse rate. You should count these pulses for one minute.

RESPIRATIONS

Respiration is the act of breathing air into the lungs (inhalation) and out of the lungs (exhalation). Oxygen is taken into the lungs during inhalation. Carbon dioxide is moved out of the lungs during exhalation. Each respiration involves one inhalation and one exhalation. The chest rises during inhalation and falls during exhalation.

The healthy adult has 14 to 20 respirations per minute. The respiratory rate is affected by many of the factors that affect body temperature and pulse rate. Heart and respiratory diseases usually cause an increased number of respirations per minute.

Abnormal respirations

Normal respirations occur between 14 and 20 times per minute in the adult. They are quiet, effortless, and regular. Both sides of the chest rise and fall equally. You should know the following abnormal respiratory patterns:

1. *Tachypnea*—rapid *(tachy)* breathing *(pnea);* the respiratory rate is usually greater than 24 respirations per minute.
2. *Bradypnea*—slow *(brady)* breathing *(pnea);* the respiratory rate is less than 10 respirations per minute.
3. *Apnea*—the lack of or absence *(a)* of breathing *(pnea)*.
4. *Hypoventilation*—respirations that are slow *(hypo)*, shallow, and sometimes irregular.
5. *Hyperventilation*—respirations that are rapid *(hyper)* and deeper than normal.
6. *Dyspnea*—difficult, labored, or painful *(dys)* breathing *(pnea)*.
7. *Cheyne-Stokes*—a breathing pattern in which respirations gradually increase in rate and depth and then become shallow and slow; breathing may stop (apnea) for 10 to 20 seconds.

Counting respirations

Respirations are counted when the resident is at rest. The resident should be positioned so you can see the chest rise and fall. The depth and rate of breathing can be voluntarily controlled to a certain extent. People tend to change breathing patterns when they know their respirations are being counted. Therefore, the resident should be unaware that respirations are being counted.

Respirations are counted right after taking a pulse. The fingers or stethoscope stay over the pulse site. The resident assumes that the pulse is still being taken. Respirations are counted by watching the rise and fall of the chest. They are counted for 30 seconds. The number is multiplied by 2 for the total number of respirations in 1 minute. If an abnormal pattern is noted, the respirations are counted for 1 full minute.

BLOOD PRESSURE

Blood pressure is the amount of force exerted against the walls of an artery by the blood. Blood pressure is controlled by the force of heart contractions, the amount of blood pumped with each heartbeat, and how easily the blood flows through the blood vessels. The period of heart muscle contraction is called *systole*. The period of heart muscle relaxation is called *diastole*.

Both the systolic and diastolic pressures are measured. The *systolic pressure* is the highest pressure. It represents the amount of force needed to pump blood out of the heart into the arteries. The *diastolic pressure* is the lowest pressure. It reflects the pressure in the arteries when the heart is at rest. Blood pressure is measured in millimeters (mm) of mercury (Hg). The systolic pressure is recorded over the diastolic pressure. The average adult has a systolic pressure of 120 mm Hg and a diastolic pressure of 80 mm Hg. This is written as 120/80 mm Hg.

Factors that affect blood pressure

Blood pressure is affected by many factors and can change from minute to minute. Age, sex, the amount of blood in the system, and emotions affect blood pressure. So do pain, exercise, body size, and medications. Because it can vary so easily, there are normal ranges for blood pressure. Systolic pressures between 100 and 150 mm Hg are normal. Normal diastolic pressures are between 60 and 90 mm Hg.

Persistent measurements above the normal systolic and diastolic pressures are abnormal. This condition is known as *hypertension*. Report any systolic pressure above 150 mm Hg to the nurse immediately. A diastolic pressure above 90 mm Hg must also be reported immediately. Likewise, systolic pressures below 100 mm Hg and diastolic pressures below 60 mm Hg are reported. This is called *hypotension*.

Some people normally have low blood pressures. However, hypotension is a sign of a serious condition that can lead to death if it is not corrected.

Equipment to measure blood pressure

A stethoscope and a sphygmomanometer are used to measure blood pressure. The *sphygmomanometer* (blood pressure cuff) consists of a cuff and a measuring device. It is sometimes called a manometer. There are three types of sphygmomanom-

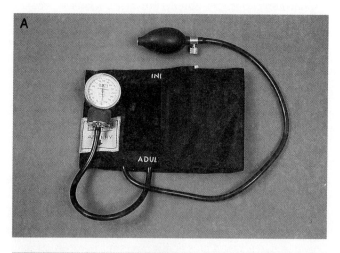

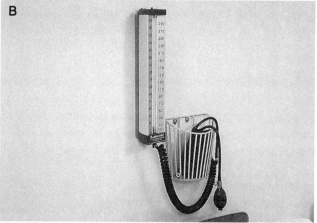

Fig. 6-16 A, Aneroid sphymomanometer and cuff. **B,** Mercury sphymomanometer and cuff. (*From Sorrentino SA:* Mosby's textbook for nursing assistants, *ed 3, St Louis, 1992, Mosby–Year Book.*)

eters: aneroid (Fig. 6-16), mercury (Fig. 6-16) and electronic (Fig. 6-17). The aneroid type has a round dial and a needle that points to the calibrations. The aneroid sphygmomanometer is small and easy to carry. The mercury sphygmomanometer is more accurate than the aneroid type. The mercury type has a column of mercury within a calibrated tube. Many facilities have wall-mounted mercury sphygmomanometers in resident rooms.

The blood pressure cuff is wrapped around the upper arm. Tubing connects the cuff to the manometer. Another tube connects the cuff to a small hand-held bulb. A valve on the bulb is turned to allow inflation of the cuff as the bulb is squeezed. The inflated cuff causes pressure over the brachial artery. The valve is turned in the opposite direction for cuff deflation. Blood pressure is measured as the cuff is deflated.

Sounds are produced as blood flows through the arteries. A stethoscope is used to hear the sounds in the brachial artery as the cuff is deflated. The first heart sound as the cuff is deflated is systolic and the last sound noted is the diastolic. Stethoscopes are not needed with electronic sphygmomanometers.

There are many types of electronic sphygmomanometers. The systolic and diastolic blood pressures are displayed on the front of the instrument. The pulse is usually displayed also. The cuff automatically inflates and deflates on some models. Others only have automatic deflation. If electronic blood pressure equipment is used where you work, you need to learn how to use the equipment. Ask the nurse to show you what to do. The manufacturer's instructions are also helpful.

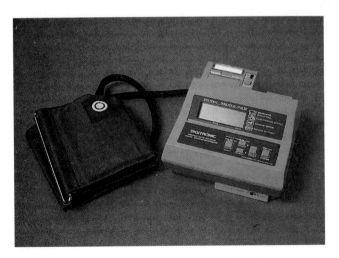

Fig. 6-17 Electronic sphymomanometer. *(From Sorrentino SA:* Mosby's textbook for nursing assistants, *ed 3, St Louis, 1992, Mosby–Year Book.)*

Measuring blood pressure

Blood pressure is normally measured in the brachial artery. You should practice the following guidelines when measuring blood pressure.

1. Blood pressure is not taken on an arm with an IV infusion or a cast, or on an arm that is injured. If a resident has had breast surgery or a stroke, blood pressure is not taken on the affected side.
2. Let the resident rest for about 15 minutes before measuring the blood pressure.
3. The cuff is applied to the bare upper arm; it is not applied over clothing. Clothing can affect the measurement.
4. The diaphragm of the stethoscope is placed firmly over the artery. The entire diaphragm must be in contact with the skin.
5. The room should be quiet so that the blood pressure can be heard. Talking, television, radio, and sounds from the hallway can make it difficult to get an accurate measurement.
6. The sphygmomanometer must be clearly visible.
7. The radial or brachial artery is located and the cuff is inflated. When the radial or brachial pulse is no longer felt, the cuff is inflated an additional 30 mm Hg. This prevents cuff inflation to a high pressure which is painful to the resident.
8. The point at which the radial pulse is no longer felt is where you should expect to hear the first blood pressure sound. The first sound is the systolic pressure. The point where the sound disappears is the diastolic pressure.

SUMMARY

Temperature, pulse, respirations, and blood pressure give valuable information about a person's health. Vital signs can vary within normal ranges. Measurements above or below a normal range signal a disorder or serious illness. Vital signs can change in response to slight changes in body functions.

Measuring vital signs is an important part of your job. Vital signs must be accurately measured. Abnormal measurements are immediately reported to the nurse. They could signal changes in a resident's condition. Clear and accurate recording of vital signs is equally important. Doctors and nurses use them to decide on treatment and to evaluate care.

CHAPTER 7

Admission and Discharge Processes

Objectives

Describe the admission process
Describe the importance of obtaining accurate weight at
    admission and at regular intervals
Measure height and weight
Record measurements accurately
Describe the discharge process

ADMISSION

Admission usually begins in an admission office. Information is gathered from the resident and family and recorded on the admission record. Information obtained includes the resident's full name, age, birthdate, physician, social security number, and religion. The resident is given an identification number. An identification band or ID picture is made.

The resident is taken to the new room, which has been prepared. The resident is greeted warmly by name. The clothing and valuables should be listed and the admission checklist completed (Fig. 7-1). Vitals signs are taken and height and weight are measured. The resident is oriented to the room and facility.

Measuring height and weight

Height and weight are measured on admission, with the resident wearing only a gown or pajamas. Shoes or slippers add weight and cause inaccurate height measurements. The person should urinate before being weighed. A full bladder can affect the weight measurement. If a urine specimen is needed, collect it at this time. The resident requiring daily weights should be weighed at the same time each day, usually before breakfast.

Standing, chair, and lift scales are available (Fig. 7-2). Chair and lift scales are used for persons who cannot stand. Follow the manufacturer's instructions when using a chair or lift scale.

Recording

Record the resident's height and weight on the admission checklist when admitting the resident. A graphic sheet or other form may be used as instructed by the nurse when additional measurements are ordered.

```
Date:_____  Time:_____  Introduced:  Self_____  Roommate_____

Admitted per:  Wheelchair_____  Cart_____  Ambulatory_____  Carried by_____

Age:_____  Sex:  M____  F____


Condition on admission:

Ambulatory      ☐     Feeds self                 ☐     Admitted by ambulance ☐     Alert      ☐
Semiambulatory  ☐     Requires help with feeding ☐     From hospital         ☐     Forgetful  ☐
Chairridden     ☐     Continent                  ☐     From home             ☐     Confused   ☐
Bedridden       ☐     Incontinent                ☐     From nursing home     ☐

State of consciousness:  Alert_____  Confused_____  Semiconscious_____  Unconscious_____

Emotional state:  Calm_____  Nervous_____  Fearful_____  Angry_____  Depressed_____

Pain:  No_____  Yes_____  Where_____

Vital signs:  BP_____  T_____  P_____  R_____  Ht_____  Wt_____

Glasses:  Yes_____  No_____  Contact lenses:  Yes_____  No_____  Hearing aid:  Yes_____  No_____

Dentures:  Yes_____  No_____  Artificial limb:  Yes_____  No_____

Artificial eye:  Yes_____  No_____  Right_____  Left_____  Pacemaker:  Yes_____  No_____

Orientation to environment:

Call light_____  Emergency light_____  Bed controls_____  Bedside stand_____  Closet_____

Drawers_____  Bathroom_____  Mealtime_____  Visiting hours_____

Information obtained from:  Patient____  Spouse_____  Parent:  M____  F____  Other_____

Other observations and comments:_____
```

Show all body marks: scars, bruises, cuts, decubiti, ulcers, and discolorations (birth marks should not be shown).

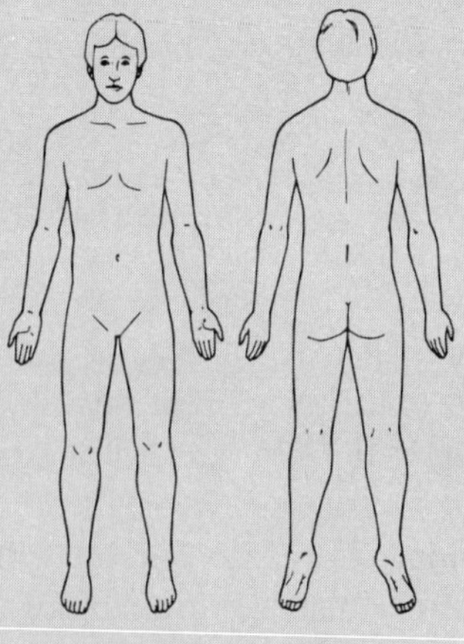

Signed _____

Fig. 7-1 Admission checklist. (*From Sorrentino SA:* Mosby's textbook for nursing assistants, *ed 3, St Louis, 1992, Mosby–Year Book.*)

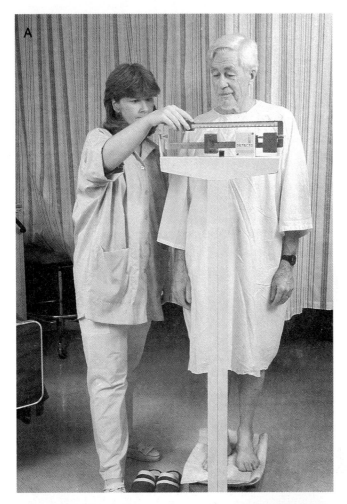

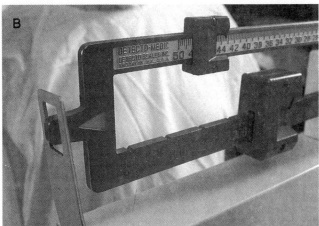

Fig. 7-2 A, The resident is being weighed. **B,** The weight is read when the balance pointer is in the middle. *(From Sorrentino SA:* Mosby's textbook for nursing assistants, *ed 3, St Louis, 1992, Mosby–Year Book.)*

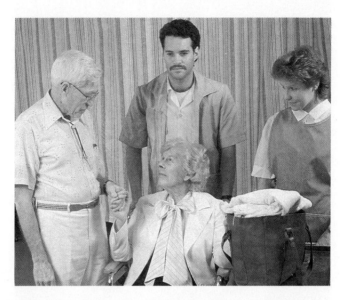

Fig. 7-3 The resident is taken to the exit by wheelchair. The resident's possessions are brought along at this time. *(From Sorrentino SA:* Mosby's textbook for nursing assistants, *ed 3, St Louis, 1992, Mosby–Year Book.)*

DISCHARGE

Discharge from a nursing facility is usually planned a few days in advance. This is a happy time if the individual is going home. Some are discharged to another hospital or to a nursing facility. Some require home care. The resident may have fears or concerns. The health team assists in planning medications, exercise, and treatments.

Nurse aides pack the resident's clothing and belongings. Valuables are returned. The nurse aide assists the resident in dressing and preparing for discharge. The health care worker assists the resident and family in transferring a resident into a car or ambulance (Fig. 7-3).

SUMMARY

Admission to a health-care facility is usually a stressful time for the resident and family. Discharge is usually happy and pleasant. However, it may cause worries and concerns if more care and treatment are required. You can help the resident and family cope with these events. You need to be polite, courteous, caring, efficient, and competent. The person's property and valuables must be handled with care and respect. They should be kept in a safe place and protected from loss or damage. Always treat the resident and family the way you would like to be treated.

CHAPTER 8

Caring for the Resident's Environment

Objectives

Identify the environmental temperature range that is comfortable for most people.

Describe how to protect residents from drafts.

Identify how to prevent or reduce odors in resident rooms.

Identify the common causes of noise in health-care facilities and how noise can be controlled.

Explain how lighting can affect the resident's comfort.

Describe the use of furniture and equipment found in a resident unit.

Describe how a bathroom is equipped for the resident's use.

Explain how to maintain the resident's unit for comfort and safety.

Describe the differences between unoccupied, open, closed, and occupied.

Identify when bed linens should be changed.

Identify the purposes of a plastic drawsheet and a cotton drawsheet.

Identify the type of bed that should be made in certain situations.

Handle linens following the rules of medical asepsis.

Residents in hospitals and long-term care facilities spend a lot of time in their rooms. Private rooms are for one person; semiprivate are furnished for two people. Rooms should be comfortable and safe. There should be enough space for the individual to perform activities of daily living. This chapter describes the conditions that influence comfort and the furnishings in a resident unit. A *resident unit* is the furniture and equipment provided for the individual by the health-care facility (Fig. 8-1).

COMFORT

Age, illness, and activity affect comfort. Comfort is also influenced by temperature, ventilation, noise, and odors. These conditions can usually be controlled to meet the person's needs.

Temperature and ventilation

Health-care facilities have heating, air conditioning, and ventilation systems. These systems maintain a comfortable temperature and provide fresh air in the rooms. A temperature range of 68° to 74° F is usually comfortable for most healthy people. A comfortable temperature for one person may be too hot or cold for another. The elderly and persons who are ill generally need higher room temperatures to be comfortable. Physically active people are usually more comfortable in cooler temperatures.

Stale room air and lingering odors cause a person to be uncomfortable and unable to rest. A good ventilation system provides fresh air and moves air in the room. Drafts can occur as air moves. The elderly and ill persons are sensitive to drafts. Protect them from drafts by having them wear enough clothing. Also make sure they are adequately covered when in bed. Move them from drafty areas whenever possible.

Odors

Many odors occur in health facilities. Some are pleasant, like food aromas and the scent of fresh flowers. Others are unpleasant. Draining wounds, vomitus, and bowel movements create unpleasant smells and can embarrass the resident. Body, breath, and smoking odors may be offensive to residents, visitors, and personnel. Ill people are usually very sensitive to odors and can become nauseated. Good ventilation helps eliminate odors. Nursing personnel can reduce odors by emptying and washing bedpans and vomit basins promptly and using room deodorizers when necessary. Good personal hygiene prevents body and breath odors.

Smoking presents special problems. Residents may be assigned to rooms on the basis of whether or not they smoke. If you smoke, do so only in designated areas. Wash your hands after handling smoking materials and before giving patient care. Careful attention must be given to your uniform, hair, and breath because of clinging smoke odors.

Many facilities ban smoking. Residents, staff, and visitors are not allowed to smoke anywhere in the building.

Noise

Elderly and ill people are sensitive to the noises and sounds around them. Residents may be easily disturbed by common health care sounds. The clanging of metal equipment such as bedpans, urinals, and wash basins and the clatter of dishes and trays may be annoying. Loud talking and laughter in hallways and at the nurse's station, loud televisions and radios, ringing telephones, and the buzzing of an intercom system can be irritating. Noise from equipment in need of repair or in need of oiling is also irritating. Wheels on stretchers, wheelchairs, utility carts, and other equipment must be oiled properly.

When in a strange place people try to figure out the cause and meaning of strange sounds. This relates to the basic need to feel safe and secure. Residents may find sounds dangerous, frightening, or irritating. As a result, they may be upset, anxious, and uncomfortable. Remember, what may not be noise to one person can be noise to another.

Health-care facilities are designed to reduce noise. Drapes, carpeting, and acoustical tiles all help absorb noise. Plastic equipment has replaced some metal equipment (for example, bedpans, urinals, and wash basins). Workers can reduce noise by controlling the loudness of their voices and by handling equipment carefully. Making sure equipment is working properly and promptly answering telephones and intercoms also decrease noise.

Lighting

Good lighting is necessary for the safety and comfort of residents and staff. Glares, shadows, and dull lighting can cause falls, headaches, and eyestrain. People usually relax and rest better when lighting is dim. However, a bright room is more cheerful and stimulating.

Lighting can be adjusted to meet the resident's changing needs. Shades can be pulled or drapes drawn to control natural light. The light above the bed can usually be adjusted to provide soft, medium, and bright lighting. Some facilities have ceiling lights over the beds. These provide very soft to extremely bright light. Bright lighting is helpful when health workers are performing procedures. Light controls should be within the resident's reach.

ROOM FURNITURE AND EQUIPMENT

Resident rooms are furnished and equipped for the person's basic needs. There is furniture and equipment for comfort, sleep, elimination, nutrition, personal hygiene, and activity (Fig. 8-1). There is also equipment in the resident's room for communicating with the nursing team, relatives, and friends. The surroundings are as homelike as possible. The right to privacy is considered when equipping the room.

The bed

Most beds in health-care facilities can be adjusted electrically or manually. They can be raised horizontally so care can be given without unnecessary bending or

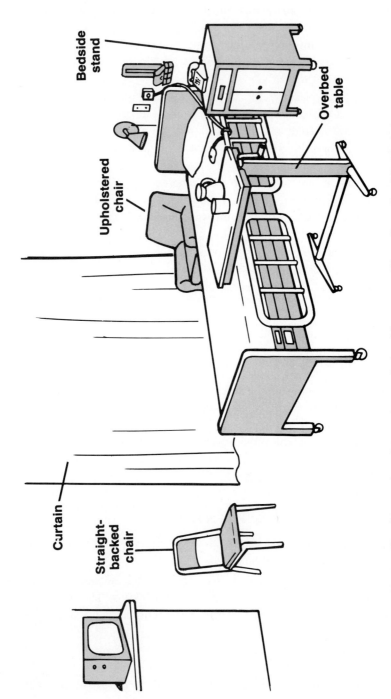

Fig. 8-1 Furniture and equipment in a typical resident room. (*From Sorrentino SA: Mosby's textbook for nursing assistants, ed 3, St Louis, 1992, Mosby–Year Book.*)

reaching. The lowest horizontal position lets the resident get out of bed with ease. The head of the bed can be kept flat or raised in varying degrees.

Electric beds are common. Bed positions are easily changed by using hand controls. The location of the controls varies with the manufacturer. They may be on a side panel, attached to the bed by a cable, or on a panel at the foot of the bed (Fig. 8-2). Residents need to know how to use the controls. They should be warned not to raise the bed to the high position and not to adjust the bed to harmful positions. They should be told if they are limited or restricted to certain positions.

Hand cranks are used to change the position of manually operated beds. The cranks are at the foot of the bed (Fig. 8-3). The left crank raises or lowers the head of the bed. The right crank adjusts the knee position. The center crank raises or lowers the entire bed horizontally. The cranks are pulled up for use and kept down at all other times. Cranks kept in the up position are safety hazards because they can be bumped into by anyone walking past them.

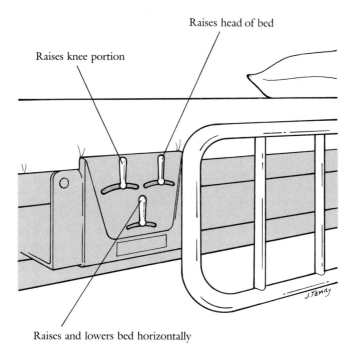

Raises head of bed

Raises knee portion

Raises and lowers bed horizontally

Fig. 8-2 Controls for an electric bed. (*From Sorrentino SA:* Mosby's textbook for nursing assistants, *ed 3, St Louis, 1992, Mosby–Year Book.*)

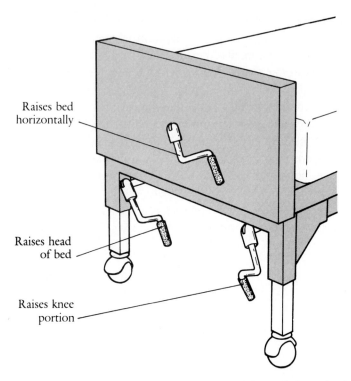

Raises bed
horizontally

Raises head
of bed

Raises knee
portion

Fig. 8-3 Manually operated hospital bed. *(From Sorrentino SA:* Mosby's textbook for nursing assistants, *ed 3, St Louis, 1992, Mosby–Year Book.)*

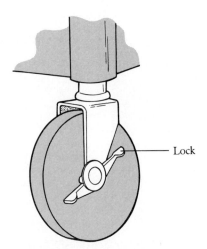

Lock

Fig. 8-4 Lock on bed wheel. *(From Sorrentino SA:* Mosby's textbook for nursing assistants, *ed 3, St Louis, 1992, Mosby–Year Book.)*

Safety considerations. Bed legs usually have wheels or casters. A *caster* is a small wheel made of rubber or plastic that allows the bed to move easily. Each wheel or caster has a lock to prevent the bed from moving (Fig. 8-4). Make sure the bed wheels are locked when giving bedside care. They should also be locked when transferring a patient to and from the bed. The patient can be injured if the bed moves.

The overbed table

The overbed table can be positioned over the bed by sliding the base under the bed. You can raise or lower the table by turning the side handle. The height can be adjusted for the resident in bed or in a chair. The overbed table is used for meal trays and for writing, reading, and other activities.

Many overbed tables have moveable tops with a storage area underneath. The storage area is often used for make-up, hair care articles, or shaving items. Many also have a flip-up mirror.

The nursing team can use the overbed table as a working area. Only *clean* and *sterile* items are placed on the table. Be sure to clean the table after using it as a working surface.

The bedside stand

The bedside stand is located next to the bed. The stand is a storage area for the resident's personal belongings and personal care equipment. It has a drawer at the top and a lower cabinet with a shelf (Fig. 8-5). The drawer can be used for small

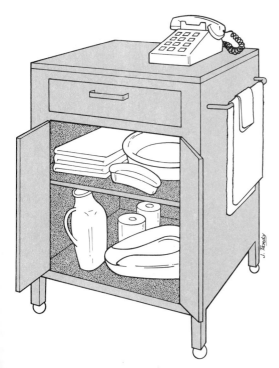

Fig. 8-5 The bedside table is used to store personal care items. *(From Sorrentino SA:* Mosby's textbook for nursing assistants, *ed 3, St Louis, 1992, Mosby–Year Book.)*

amounts of money, eyeglasses, books, and other personal possessions. The first shelf is used for the wash basin, which can hold personal care items. These include soap, soap dish, powder, lotion, deodorant, towels, washcloth, bath blanket, and a clean gown or pajamas. A vomit or kidney basin is often used to hold oral hygiene equipment. The kidney basin can be stored in the top shelf or in the drawer. The bedpan and its cover, the urinal, and toilet paper are kept on the lower shelf. This prevents the spread of germs.

The top stand is often used for tissues and the telephone. The top may also be used for a radio, flowers, gifts, cards, and other items important to the patient. Some stands have a rod at the side or back for towels and washcloths.

Chairs

The resident's room usually has at least two chairs. One is a straight-backed chair with no arms and the other an upholstered chair with arms. The upholstered chair is used most often by the resident and visitors. It is placed near the bed. Some facilities allow residents to bring a favorite chair from home.

Curtains or screens

Semiprivate rooms have a curtain between the two residents. The curtain can be pulled around either bed to provide privacy. The curtain is always pulled while care is being given. If a portable screen is used (Fig. 8-6), it is placed between the two beds. Curtains and screens protect the resident's privacy. However, they do not block sound or prevent conversations from being heard.

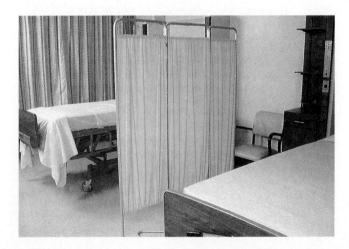

Fig. 8-6 Portable screen. (*From Sorrentino SA:* Mosby's textbook for nursing assistants, *ed 3, St Louis, 1992, Mosby–Year Book.*)

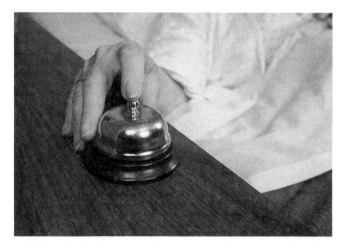

Fig. 8-7 Tap bell. *(From Sorrentino SA:* Mosby's textbook for nursing assistants, *ed 3, St Louis, 1992, Mosby–Year Book.)*

Personal care equipment

Personal care equipment refers to the items needed for hygiene and elimination. It usually includes a wash basin, vomit or kidney basin, bedpan, urinal, water pitcher, drinking glass, soap, and soap dish. Powder, lotion, toothbrush, toothpaste, mouthwash, tissues, and a comb may also be provided. Residents usually bring their own oral hygiene equipment, hair care supplies, and deodorant. Some choose to use their own soap, lotion, and powder.

Call system

The call system lets the resident signal when help is needed. A signal light at the bedside is connected to a light above the room door and to a light panel or intercom system at the nurse's station. The signal light is at the end of a long cord. It can be attached to the bed or chair so that it is always within the resident's reach. The patient presses a button at the end of the signal light when assistance is needed. The nurse or nurse aide shuts off the light at the bedside when the resident is given the help needed.

Some facilities have intercom systems that allow members of the nursing team to talk with the resident from the nurse's station. It also allows the light to be shut off from the station. A tap bell is sometimes used in place of the signal light (Fig. 8-7). The signal light or tap bell must always be within reach. Residents are shown how to use the call system when admitted to the facility.

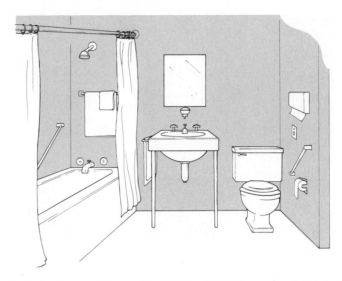

Fig. 8-8 Resident's bathroom in a nursing facility. (*From Sorrentino SA:* Mosby's textbook for nursing assistants, *ed 3, St Louis, 1992, Mosby–Year Book.*)

The bathroom

Many health-care facilities have a bathroom in each room. Some have a bathroom between two resident rooms. A toilet, sink, call system, and mirror are standard equipment. Some bathrooms are equipped with a tub and shower (Fig. 8-8) or with just a shower. Hand rails, which can be used by the patient for support, are installed by the toilet. Toilets in some facilities are higher than the standard toilet. The higher toilets make transfers from wheelchairs to toilets easier and are helpful for residents with joint problems.

Towel racks, toilet paper, soap, a paper towel dispenser, and the call system are found in the bathroom. They are placed within easy reach of the resident.

Closet and drawer space

Most hospitals provide closet and extra drawer space for the resident's clothing. OBRA requires nursing facilities to provide each resident with closet space, which must have shelves and a clothes rack. The resident must have free access to the closet and its contents.

Items in the closet or drawers are the person's private property. You must not search the closet or drawers without the person's permission.

Sometimes people "hoard" items like napkins, straws, sugar, salt, pepper, and food in their drawers. Such hoarding can cause safety and health risks. Facilities can inspect a person's closet or drawers if hoarding is suspected. The person must be informed of the inspection and be in the room when it takes place.

Other equipment

Many facilities furnish resident rooms with additional equipment. A television and radio are often included for comfort and relaxation, along with a telephone for talking to family and friends. A wastebasket is placed by the bed.

In some facilities blood pressure equipment is often mounted on walls. There are also wall outlets for oxygen and suction. An IV pole (IV standard) is used to hang an IV infusion bottle or bag. Some beds have an IV pole stored in the bedframe. The IV pole may be a separate piece of equipment that is brought to the room as needed.

GENERAL RULES

The resident's room must be kept clean, neat, and safe. This is a responsibility of everyone involved in the person's care. The following rules will help guide you in maintaining the resident's environment.

1. Arrange personal belongings as the resident prefers. Make sure they are easily reached.
2. Keep the signal light within the resident's reach at all times.
3. Make sure the resident can reach the telephone, television controls, and light controls.
4. Adjust lighting, temperature, and ventilation for the resident's comfort.
5. Handle equipment carefully to prevent unnecessary noise.
6. Explain the causes of strange noises to the patient.
7. Use room deodorizers if necessary.
8. Empty the resident's wastebasket as often as needed.
9. Keep the bed locked in the lowest position, except when providing resident care.
10. Keep side rails up while the resident is in bed.
11. After each use, clean resident equipment and return it to its storage place.

Bedmaking

Residents spend a lot of time in bed. Some are out of bed part of the day, while others must be in bed all the time. Meals are eaten in bed and some residents are bathed in bed. Some cannot get out of bed to use the bathroom. Many treatments are done with the resident in bed.

Bedmaking is an important part of your job. A clean and neat bed helps make you resident more comfortable.

Beds are usually made in the morning after baths. The bed can also be made while the resident is in the shower, tub, or out of the room.

Linens are straightened if they become loose and wrinkled during the day. Check linens for crumbs after meals and remove them. Be sure to straighten linens at bedtime. You must change linens if they become wet, soiled, or damp.

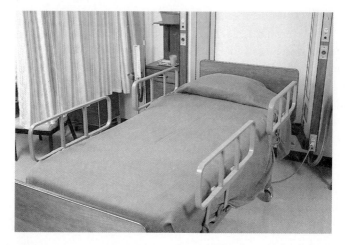

Fig. 8-9 A closed bed. *(From Sorrentino SA:* Mosby's textbook for nursing assistants, *ed 3, St Louis, 1992, Mosby–Year Book.)*

Beds are made in the following ways.

1. A *closed bed* is one where the top linens are not folded back (Fig. 8-9).
2. An *open bed* is being used by a resident. Top linens are folded back so that the resident can easily get into bed. A closed bed becomes an open bed by folding back the top linens (Fig. 8-10).
3. An *occupied bed* is made with the resident in it (Fig. 8-11).

LINENS

Special attention is given to the care and use of linens. The rules of medical asepsis are followed when handling linens and making beds. Your uniform is considered to be dirty, so always hold linens away from your body and uniform. Never shake linens in the air. Shaking them causes the spread of microorganisms. Clean linens are placed on a clean surface. Never put dirty linen on the floor.

Linens are collected in the order they will be used. Do not bring extra linens to a resident's room. Extra linen in a room is considered to be contaminated and cannot be used for another resident.

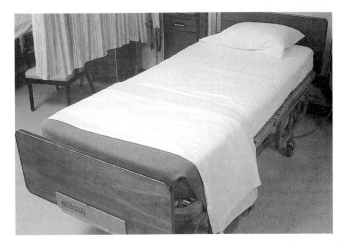

Fig. 8-10 An open bed. *(From Sorrentino SA:* Mosby's textbook for nursing assistants, *ed 3, St Louis, 1992, Mosby–Year Book.)*

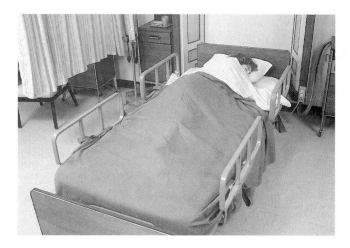

Fig. 8-11 An occupied bed. *(From Sorrentino SA:* Mosby's textbook for nursing assistants, *ed 3, St Louis, 1992, Mosby–Year Book.)*

You should collect the following and place them in order that they will be used.

1. Bath blanket
2. Gown or clothes
3. Washcloth
4. Hand towel
5. Bath towel(s)
6. Mattress pad
7. Bottom sheet (flat sheet or contour sheet)
8. Plastic drawsheet or rubber drawsheet
9. Cotton drawsheet
10. Top sheet (flat sheet)
11. Blanket
12. Bedspread
13. Pillowcase(s)

A *bath blanket* is a thin, lightweight cotton blanket used to cover the resident during a bath or other procedures. It absorbs moisture and provides warmth.

Linens are pressed and folded to prevent the spread of microbes and for easy bedmaking. They are pressed with a center crease which is placed in the center of the bed from the head to the foot. The linens unfold easily.

To remove dirty linen from the bed, roll the linens up away from you. The side that touched the resident is inside the roll. The side that has not touched the resident is outside (Fig. 8-12).

Not all linens are changed every time the bed is made. Some are reused for an open or closed bed. The mattress pad, plastic drawsheet, blanket, and bedspread may be reused for the same resident. They can be reused if not soiled, wet, or very wrinkled. Some facilities use only flat sheets. The flat top sheet can be reused as the bottom sheet. If a resident has been discharged, all linens are removed and a closed bed is made. Check the facility's policy about linen changes. *Remember, linens that are wet, damp, or soiled must be changed right away.*

A standard bed includes a rubber or plastic drawsheet and a cotton drawsheet. A *drawsheet* is a small sheet placed over the middle of the bottom sheet. It helps keep the mattress and bottom linens clean and dry. A *plastic* or *rubber drawsheet* protects the mattress and bottom linens from becoming damp or soiled. It is placed between the bottom sheet and cotton drawsheet. The cotton drawsheet is needed to protect the resident from contact with the plastic or rubber and to absorb moisture. Although the bottom linen and mattress were protected, resident discomfort and skin breakdown are occasionally noted. These are due to heat retention and the difficulty in keeping the drawsheets tight and wrinkle free.

Most mattresses made for clinical use are covered with plastic. Plastic mattress

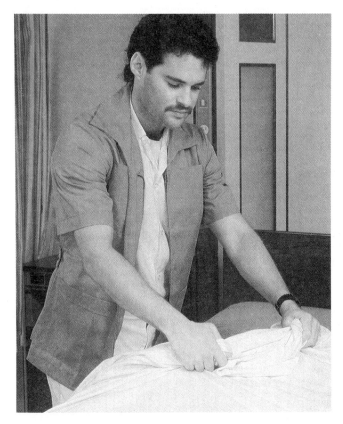

Fig. 8-12 Roll linens away from you when removing them from a bed. *(From Sorrentino SA: Mosby's textbook for nursing assistants, ed 3, St Louis, 1992, Mosby–Year Book.)*

covers can be used. Disposable waterproof bed protectors can also be used. Plastic and cotton drawsheets may be reserved for certain residents. They include those with bowel- or bladder-control problems or those who have excessive wound drainage.

A cotton drawsheet may be used without a plastic drawsheet. Plasticized mattresses cause some residents to perspire heavily and increases their discomfort. A cotton drawsheet helps reduce heat retention and absorbs moisture. Cotton drawsheets are often used as lift sheets to move and position residents in bed. When used for this purpose, they are not tucked in at the sides. The bedmaking procedures in this chapter include plastic and cotton drawsheets. Consult the nurse about their use. Also, know your facility's policies about using plastic and cotton drawsheets.

BEDMAKING
General rules

Remember these rules when making a resident's bed.

1. Use good body mechanics at all times.
2. Follow the rules of medical asepsis.
3. Always wash your hands before handling clean linen and after handling dirty linen.
4. Bring enough linen to the resident's room.
5. Never shake linens. Shaking linens cause the spread of microorganisms.
6. Extra linen in a resident's room is considered contaminated. Put it in the dirty laundry so it is not used for other residents.
7. Hold linens away from your uniform. Dirty and clean linen should never touch your uniform.
8. Never put dirty linen on the floor or on clean linens. Follow facility policy about dirty linen.
9. Linens, especially bottom linens, should be tight and free of wrinkles.
10. A cotton drawsheet must completely cover the plastic drawsheet. A plastic drawsheet should never touch the resident's body.
11. Straighten and tighten loose sheets, blankets, and bedspreads whenever necessary.
12. Make as much of one side of the bed as possible before going to the other side. This saves time and energy.

A *closed* bed is made after a resident has been discharged so that it is ready for a new resident. The bed is made after the bed frame and mattress have been cleaned according to the facility's policy.

The *open* bed is an unoccupied bed. Linens are folded back so the resident can get into bed with ease. Open beds are made when residents are admitted to the facility. They are also made for residents who can be out of bed when their beds are being made. A closed bed easily becomes an open bed by folding back the top linens.

An occupied bed is made when a resident cannot get out of bed because of illness or injury. When making an occupied bed you must keep the resident in good body alignment. You must also be aware of restrictions or limitations in the resident's movement or positioning. Be sure to explain each step of the procedure to the resident before it is done.

Procedures
1. Wash your hands.
2. Gather linen and place in order on a bedside chair.

3. Introduce yourself to the resident and provide for privacy (when making an occupied bed).
4. Raise the bed to the highest level.
5. Lower the head of the bed. Remove the pillow and pillowcase.
6. Lower the side rail.
7. Roll top linens into a bundle and place in linen bag (when making an occupied bed, place a bath blanket over the resident first).
8. Loosen and remove bottom linens by rolling them into the center.
9. Place the mattress pad on the bed.
10. Place the bottom sheet on the bed lengthwise and roll in towards center. (If flat sheet used, make a corner at top of sheet and tuck under mattress lengthwise to foot of bed.)
11. Place rubber drawsheet and cotton drawsheet on bed; fan fold to the center.
12. Apply top lines, sheet, and bedspread lengthwise; make a corner with sheet at foot of bed. (When making an occupied bed, pull the side rail up before going to the opposite side of the bed).
13. Remove the soiled bottom linen and place it in laundry bag.
14. Straighten mattress pad.
15. Pull bottom sheet through, make mitered corner at head of bed, and tuck sheet under mattress (head to foot).
16. Bring top linens across resident; remove bath blanket from the resident in an occupied bed; tuck the linens under the foot of the bed, miter the corner.
17. Make a cuff at top of bed by bringing top sheet over bedspread.
18. Place pillowcase on a pillow.
19. Place bed in the lowest position.

SUMMARY

The resident's room is designed and equipped to meet basic needs. Equipment is provided for comfort, hygiene, elimination, and activity. The overbed table is used for self-care activities and resident care. Side rails, hand rails, and the call system are for resident safety. Keep the side rails up and the bed in its lowest position. Safety is also promoted by controlling temperature, ventilation, lighting, noise, and odors. Curtains or screens provide privacy and also help the resident feel safe and secure. A telephone lets the resident talk with family and friends. The television and radio provide entertainment and relaxation.

You have learned how to make beds for different resident needs. You have also learned the principles of bedmaking and of handling linens. The resident's comfort and safety are the focus of bedmaking. Remember that the resident spends a lot of time in bed. Therefore, the bed must be neat, clean, and free of wrinkles. A well-made bed helps make your resident more comfortable.

CHAPTER 9

Recognizing Abnormal Signs and Symptoms of Common Diseases

Objectives

Describe glaucoma, cataracts, and measures for dealing with the blind.

Describe how to communicate with the hearing impaired.

Identify the causes and effects of head and spinal cord injuries and the care required.

Define hemiplegia, paraplegia, and quadriplegia.

Discuss gastrointestinal changes that occur with age.

Identify reproductive system changes that occur with age.

Explain how to maintain joint function in arthritis.

Explain how to care for patients in casts, in traction, and with hip pinnings.

Describe osteoporosis and the care required.

Explain why loss of a limb requires a major psychological adjustment.

List the risk factors for coronary artery disease.

Describe angina pectoris, myocardial infarction, congestive heart failure, and the care required.

Identify the signs, symptoms, complications, and treatment of hypertension.

Describe common respiratory disorders and care required.

Identify the signs, symptoms, and complications of diabetes mellitus.

Describe AIDS and hepatitis, their signs and symptoms, and necessary precautions.

Describe a cerebrovascular accident, its signs and symptoms, and the care required.

Describe Parkinson's disease and multiple sclerosis.

Describe changes that occur in the urinary system as a result of aging or injury.

Identify the warning signs of cancer and how cancer is treated.

Many residents in nursing facilities have health disorders. Basic information about common disorders and diseases are presented in this chapter. Having basic information about these disorders makes the required care more meaningful. If more information is needed, the nurse aide should ask the charge nurse for additional explanation.

VISION PROBLEMS

Vision problems occur at all ages. Problems range from very mild loss to complete blindness. They may be sudden or gradual in onset. One or both eyes may be affected. Surgery, eyeglasses, or contact lenses are often necessary.

Glaucoma

Glaucoma is an eye disorder. Pressure within the eye is increased, which damages the retina and optic nerve. The result is visual loss with eventual blindness. The disease may be gradual or sudden in onset. Signs and symptoms include tunnel vision (Fig. 9-1), blurred vision, and blue-green halos around lights. With sudden onset, the patient also has severe eye pain, nausea, and vomiting. Glaucoma is a major cause of blindness. Persons over 40 years of age are at risk. The cause is unknown.

Treatment involves drug therapy and possibly surgery. The goal is to prevent further damage to the retina and optic nerve. Damage that has already occurred cannot be reversed.

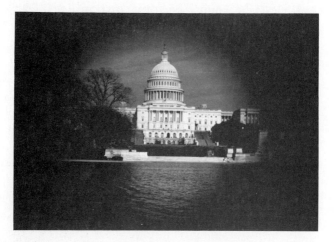

Fig. 9-1 Tunnel vision. (*From Sorrentino SA:* Mosby's textbook for nursing assistants, *ed 3, St Louis, 1992, Mosby-Year Book.*)

Cataracts

A cataract is an eye disorder in which the lens becomes cloudy (opaque). The cloudiness prevents light from entering the eye. Gradual blurring and dimming of vision occurs. Sight is eventually lost. A cataract can occur in one or both eyes. Aging is the most common cause. Surgery is the only treatment.

The resident may have to wear an eye shield or patch for several days after surgery. The shield protects the eye from injury. One or both eyes may be covered. Measures for the blind person are practiced when an eye shield is worn. Even if only one shield is worn, the person is still at risk since there may be visual loss in the other eye from a cataract or other causes.

The resident is fitted with corrective lenses after surgery. A permanent implant may be done during surgery. Even with corrective lenses or implants, there will be some degree of impaired vision.

Corrective lenses

Eyeglasses and contact lenses are prescribed to correct vision problems. Eyeglasses may be worn only for certain activities, such as reading or seeing at a distance. They may also be worn continuously while awake. Contact lenses are usually worn continuously while awake.

Eyeglasses. The person may be upset when glasses are first needed. However, adjustment is usually rapid. Most people accept the fact that they will need glasses sooner or later.

Lenses are made of hardened glass or plastic. They are impact resistant to prevent shattering. Glass lenses are washed with warm water and dried with soft tissue. Plastic lenses are easily scratched. A special cleaning solution and special tissues and cloths are needed for cleaning and drying them.

Glasses are costly. They must be protected from breakage or other damage. When not being worn, they need to be put in their case. The case is put in the drawer of the bedside stand. Glasses are easily damaged or lost if not in the case and in the drawer.

Contact lenses. Contact lenses fit directly on the eye. Hard and soft contacts are available. Many people prefer contacts because they cannot be seen. They do not break easily, and can be worn for sports. However, contacts are more expensive than eyeglasses. They are also easily lost. Contacts are removed for activities like swimming, showering, and sleeping.

Persons with contact lenses are taught to insert, remove, and clean them. Residents should perform these activities personally. However, a resident may be unable to insert or remove the lenses. A nurse is responsible for meeting these resident's needs. The eye can easily be damaged when inserting or removing contact lenses. Therefore, you should not perform these measures.

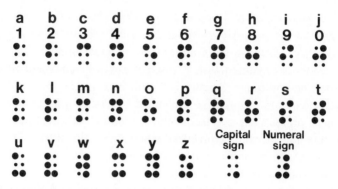

Fig. 9-2 Braille. *(From Sorrentino SA:* Mosby's textbook for nursing assistants, *ed 3, St Louis, 1992, Mosby–Year Book.)*

Blindness

Blindness has many causes. Birth defects, accidents, and eye diseases are examples. It can also be a complication of diseases that affect other organs and body systems. Blindness is usually acquired later in life. A person's life is seriously affected by the loss of sight. Physical and psychological adjustments can be long and difficult. Special education and training are required. Moving about, activities of daily living, reading braille, and using a seeing-eye dog require training.

Braille is a method of writing for the blind that uses raised dots. The dots are arranged to represent each letter of the alphabet. The first 10 letters also represent the numbers 0 through 9 (Fig. 9-2). The person feels the arrangement of the dots with the fingers. Many books, magazines, and newspapers are available in braille. There are also braille typewriters.

Braille is hard to learn, especially for many elderly people. Therefore, books and other reading materials are available on records and tapes. These are often called "talking books." They can be bought or borrowed from libraries.

The blind person can be taught to move about with a white cane or a seeing-eye (guide) dog. Both are recognized worldwide as signs that the person is blind. The dog serves as the eyes of the blind person. The dog recognizes danger and guides the person on sidewalks.

You must treat a blind person with respect and dignity—not pity. Most blind people have adjusted to their blindness. They lead rather independent lives. Certain practices are necessary when dealing with a blind person. These practices are necessary no matter how long the person has been blind.

1. Identify yourself promptly when you enter the room. Give your name, title, and reason for being there. Do not touch the person until you have indicated your presence in the room.
2. Orient the person to the room. Identify the location and purpose of furniture and equipment.
3. Allow the person to touch and locate furniture and equipment if able.
4. Do not rearrange furniture and equipment.
5. Give step-by-step explanations of procedures as you perform them. Indicate when the procedure is over.
6. Tell the person when you are leaving the room.
7. Keep doors open or shut, never partially open.
8. Help the person walk by walking slightly ahead of him or her. The person should touch your arm lightly. *Never* push or guide the blind person in front of you.
9. Inform the person of steps, doors, turns, furniture, curbs, and other obstructions when assisting with walking.
10. Assist in food selection by reading the menu to the person.
11. Explain the location of food and beverages on the tray. Use an imaginary clock or guide the person's hand to each item on the tray.
12. Cut up meat, open containers, butter bread, and other similiar activities if needed.
13. Keep the signal light within the resident's reach.
14. Provide a radio, "talking books," television, and braille books for the resident's entertainment.
15. Do not shout or speak in a loud voice. Just because a person is blind does not mean that hearing is impaired.
16. Let the person perform self-care activities if able.

HEARING PROBLEMS

Hearing losses range from slight hearing impairments to complete deafness. Hearing is required for many functions. Talking, responsiveness to others, safety, and awareness of surroundings all require hearing. Many people deny that it is difficult for them to hear well. This is because hearing loss is usually associated with aging.

Effects on the resident

A person may be unaware of gradual difficulty in hearing. Families or friends may notice changes in the person's behavior or attitude. However, they may not realize that the changes are due to hearing difficulties. The symptoms and effects of hearing loss vary. They are not always obvious to the person or to others.

There are obvious signs of hearing impairment. These include speaking too loudly, leaning forward to hear, and turning and cupping the better ear toward the speaker. The person may respond the wrong way or ask for words to be repeated.

Psychological and social effects are less obvious. People with hearing problems may tend to avoid social situations. This is an attempt to avoid embarrassment, but loneliness, boredom, and feelings of being left out often result. Only parts of conversations may be heard. People with hearing loss become suspicious if they think they are being talked about or that others are talking softly on purpose. Some try to talk too much so that they do not have to respond or answer questions. Straining and working hard to hear can cause fatigue, frustration, and irritability.

People with hearing loss may develop speech problems. You hear yourself as you talk. How you pronounce words and your voice volume depend on how you hear yourself. Hearing loss may result in slurred speech and improper word pronunciation. Monotone speech and dropping word endings may also occur.

Communicating with the resident

Hearing-impaired persons may wear hearing aids or read lips. They also watch facial expressions, gestures, and body language to understand what is being said. Sign language may be necessary for the totally deaf. Some hearing-impaired people have "hearing" dogs. The dogs alert the person to such things as ringing phones, door bells, sirens, or on-coming cars. Certain measures are necessary when communicating with the person with a hearing loss. The following measures can help the person hear or lip read.

1. Gain attention and alert the person to your presence in the room by lightly touching their arm. Do not startle or approach the person from behind.
2. Face the person directly when speaking. Do not turn or walk away while you are talking.
3. Stand or sit in good light. Shadows and glares affect the person's ability to see your face clearly.
4. Speak clearly, distinctly, and slowly.
5. Speak in a normal tone of voice. Do not shout.
6. Do not cover your mouth, smoke, eat, or chew gum while talking. They affect mouth movements.
7. State the topic of conversation or discussion first.
8. Use short sentences and simple words.
9. Write out important names.
10. Keep conversations and discussions short to avoid tiring the person.
11. Repeat and rephrase statements as needed.

12. Be alert to the messages sent by your facial expressions, gestures, and body language.
13. Reduce or eliminate background noises.

The person with a hearing impairment may have speech problems. Understanding what the person is saying can be difficult. Make sure that you understand what is being said. Do not pretend to understand to avoid the person's embarrassment. Serious consequences can result if you assume or pretend to understand. The following guidelines will help you to communicate with the speech-impaired person.

1. Listen and give the person your full attention.
2. Ask the person questions to which you know the answer. This helps you to become familiar with the person's speech.
3. Determine the subject being discussed. This helps you understand essential points.
4. Ask the person to repeat or rephrase statements if necessary.
5. Repeat what the person has said. Ask if you have understood correctly.
6. Ask the person to write down key words or the message if necessary.
7. Watch the person's lip movements.
8. Watch facial expressions, gestures, and body language for clues about what is being said.

Hearing aids

A *hearing aid* makes sounds louder. It does not correct or cure the hearing problem. The actual ability to hear is not improved. Both background noise and speech are made louder. Noise must be reduced to help the person adjust to the hearing aid. Remember that a hearing aid does not make speech clearer, only louder. The measures for communicating with hearing-impaired persons apply to those with hearing aids.

Hearing aids are operated by batteries. There is an on and off switch. Sometimes hearing aids do not work properly. Several things need to be checked. Determine if the instrument is on or off. Proper battery position also needs to be checked. New batteries may be needed. The earpiece may need cleaning, or the hearing aid may need repair.

Hearing aids are expensive. They must be handled carefully and cared for properly. The earpiece (Fig. 9-3) is the only part that can be washed. Soap and water are used daily to wash the hearing aid. Thorough drying of the earpiece is necessary before it is snapped back into place.

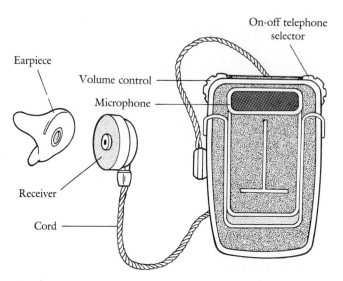

Fig. 9-3 Parts of a hearing aid. (*From Sorrentino SA:* Mosby's textbook for nursing assistants, *ed 3, St Louis, 1992, Mosby–Year Book.)*

HEAD INJURIES

Blows to the scalp and skull may cause brain tissue to be injured. Sometimes injuries are minor. Minor injuries may cause only a temporary loss of consciousness. Others are more serious. Permanent brain damage or death may result. Brain tissue can be bruised or torn. Skull fractures can cause brain damage. Bleeding from head injuries can occur in the brain or surrounding structures.

Head injuries are caused by many things, including falls, car accidents, industrial accidents, and sports injuries. Other body parts may be injured also, such as the spinal cord. Birth injuries are another major cause of head trauma. If the person survives a severe head injury, some permanent damage is likely. Paralysis, mental retardation, personality changes, speech problems, breathing difficulties, and loss of bowel and bladder control may be permanent. Rehabilitation is required. Nursing care depends on the resident's needs and remaining abilities.

SPINAL CORD INJURIES

Spinal cord injuries can permanently damage the nervous system. These injuries usually occur from stab or bullet wounds, vehicle accidents, industrial accidents, falls, or sports injuries.

The type of damage depends on the area injured. If the injury is in the lumbar area, muscle function in the legs is lost. Injuries at the thoracic level cause loss of muscle function below the chest. Residents with injuries at the lumbar or thoracic levels are paraplegics. *Paraplegia* is paralysis of the legs. Cervical injuries may result in loss of function to the arms, chest, and all muscles below the chest. Residents with these injuries are quadriplegics. *Quadriplegia* is paralysis of the arms, legs, and trunk.

If the person survives, rehabilitation is necessary. The resident's needs and the rehabilitation program depend on the functions lost and the remaining abilities. Emotional needs cannot be overlooked. These persons have severe emotional reactions to paralysis and the loss of function. Paralyzed residents generally need the following care.

1. Protect the resident from injury. Falls and burns are major risks. Keep side rails up, the bed in the low position, and the call light within reach. Bath water, heat applications, and food must be at the proper temperature.
2. Turn and reposition the resident every 2 hours.
3. Give skin care and other measures to prevent decubitus ulcers.
4. Maintain good body alignment at all times. Pillows, trochanter rolls, foot boards, and other devices are used as needed.
5. Carry out bowel and bladder training programs.
6. Perform range-of-motion exercises to maintain muscle function and prevent contractures. Other exercises may be ordered.
7. Assist with food and fluids as needed. The resident may have to be fed. Self-help devices may be needed.
8. Give emotional and psychological support. Mental health specialists may be involved in the care.
9. Physical therapy, occupational therapy, and vocational rehabilitation may be ordered. They help the resident regain independent functioning as much as possible.

GASTROINTESTINAL SYSTEM CHANGES

Many changes affect the gastrointestinal (digestive) system in the elderly. Difficulty in swallowing (dysphagia) often occurs due to certain medical conditions or decreases in the amount of saliva. Taste and smell become dulled, causing a decrease in appetite. Secretion of digestive juices decreases. As a result, fried and fatty foods are difficult to digest and cause indigestion. Loss of teeth and ill-fitting dentures make chewing difficult. This results in digestion problems. Decreased peristalsis results in slower emptying of the stomach and colon. Gas and constipation are common because of decreased peristalsis. Dry, fried, and fatty foods should be avoided. This helps avoid the problems of difficulty in swallowing and indigestion. Good oral hygiene and denture care helps the ability to taste. People may not have natural teeth or dentures. Their food has to be pureed or ground. Avoiding high-fiber foods may be necessary even though they help prevent constipation. Foods high in fiber are difficult to chew and can irritate the intestines. High-fiber foods include apricots, celery, and fruits and vegetables with skins and seeds. Foods that provide soft bulk are often ordered for those with chewing difficulties or constipation. These foods include whole-grain cereals and cooked fruits and vegetables.

Aging requires dietary changes. Elderly people need fewer calories than younger people. Energy levels and daily activity levels are lower. Additional fluids are needed to promote kidney function. Foods that prevent constipation and musculoskeletal changes need to be included in the diet. The diet should also include enough protein for tissue growth and repair. However, protein may be lacking in the diets of the elderly as foods high in protein are generally the most expensive.

REPRODUCTIVE SYSTEM

The organs of reproduction change during the aging process. Changes do not eliminate sexual needs or abilities. Changes in the male are related to decreases in the hormone testosterone. This hormone affects strength, sperm production, and reproductive tissues. Changes in sexual activity are related to erections. It takes longer for an erection to occur and there is a longer time period between erection and ejaculation.

Physical changes also occur in women. Menopause, when menstruation stops, occurs in women around 50 years of age. There is a decreased secretion of the female hormones (estrogen and progesterone). The uterus, vagina, and external genitals decrease in size. The woman experiences thinning of vaginal walls and decreased secretions, which may cause discomfort during intercourse.

MUSCULOSKELETAL SYSTEM

As aging progresses, there is gradual muscle atrophy (shrinking) and decreasing strength. Bones become brittle and can break easily. Joints become stiff and painful. These changes result in a gradual loss of height, loss of strength, and decreased mobility. There is the possibility of a fracture (broken bone) from simply turning in bed.

To help slow down this process, encourage the person to be as active as possible. This should include range-of-motion exercises and good nutrition. The diet should be high in protein, calcium, and vitamins. Because bones can break easily, the individual must be protected from injury. Measures to prevent falls must be practiced. The individual is turned and moved gently and carefully. A person may need support and assistance when getting out of bed and when walking. A cane or walker may be needed.

Arthritis means joint *(arth)* inflammation *(itis)*. It is the most common joint disease. Pain and decreased mobility occur in the affected joints. There are two basic types of arthritis.

Osteoarthritis occurs with aging. Joint injury is also a cause. The hips and knees are commonly affected. These joints bear the weight of the body. Joints in the fingers, thumbs, and spine can also be affected. Symptoms are joint stiffness and pain. Cold weather and dampness seem to increase the symptoms.

Osteoarthritis has no cure. Treatment involves relieving pain and stiffness. Doctors often order aspirin for the pain. Local heat applications may be ordered. When the condition is advanced, the resident may need help walking.

Rheumatoid arthritis is a chronic disease. It can occur at any age. Connective tissue throughout the body is affected. The disease affects the heart, lungs, eyes, kidneys, and skin. However, mainly the joints are affected. Smaller joints in the fingers, hands, and wrists are affected first. Larger joints are eventually involved. Severe inflammation causes very painful and swollen joints. The pain will probably restrict body movements.

Signs and symptoms are: pain, redness, and swelling in the joint area; limitation of joint motion; fever; fatigue; and weight loss. As the disease progresses, more and more joints become involved. Changes in other organs eventually occur.

The goals in treating rheumatoid arthritis are:

1. Maintaining joint motion
2. Controlling pain
3. Preventing deformities

The resident needs a lot of rest. Bed rest may be ordered if several joints are involved and when fever is present. If the resident is prescribed bed rest, turning and repositioning are done every 2 hours. The resident is positioned to prevent contractures. Eight to 10 hours of sleep are needed each night. Morning and afternoon rest periods are also necessary. Rest is balanced with exercise. Range-of-motion exercises are done. Walking aids may be needed. Splints may be applied to the affected body parts. Nurse aides need to follow the splint schedule. Safety measures to prevent falls are practiced.

Medications are ordered by the doctor for pain. Local heat applications may be ordered, and a back massage is often relaxing. Positioning to prevent deformities promotes comfort.

Residents need emotional support and reassurance. The disease is chronic. Death from other organ involvement is possible. A good attitude is important. Residents should be as active as possible. Encourage them to do as much self-care as possible.

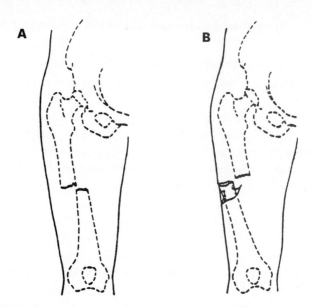

Fig. 9-4. A, Closed fracture. **B,** Open fracture. *(From Harkness-Hood GH, Dincher JR: Total patient care: foundations and practices, ed 7, St Louis, 1988, Mosby–Year Book.)*

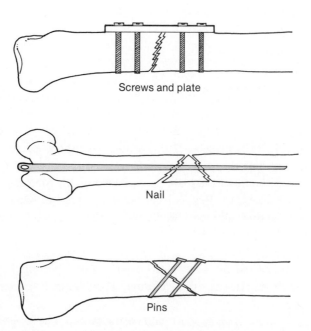

Screws and plate

Nail

Pins

Fig. 9-5. Devices used to reduce a fracture. *(From Miliken ME, Campbell G: Essential competencies for patient care, St Louis, 1985, Mosby–Year Book.)*

Fractures

A *fracture* is a broken bone. Tissues around the fracture (muscles, blood vessels, nerves, and tendons) are usually injured also. Fractures may be open or closed (Fig. 9-4). A *closed fracture (simple fracture)* means the bone is broken but the skin is intact. An *open fracture (compound fracture)* means the broken bone has come through the skin.

Fractures are caused by falls and accidents. A bone disease called osteoporosis can also lead to fractures. Signs and symptoms of a fracture are pain, swelling, limitation of movement, bruising, and color changes at the fracture site. Bleeding may occur.

The bone has to heal. The two bone ends are brought back into normal position. This is called reduction. *Closed reduction* involves manipulating the bone back into place. The skin is not opened. *Open reduction* involves surgery. The bone is exposed and brought back into alignment. Nails, pins, screws, metal plates, or wires may be used to keep the bones in place (Fig. 9-5). After reduction, the fracture is immobilized. In other words, movement of the two bone ends is prevented. A cast or traction may be used to keep the bone from moving.

Cast care. Casts are made of plaster of paris, plastic, or fiber glass. The cast covers all or part of an extremity. A plaster of paris cast needs 24 to 48 hours to dry. A dry cast is odorless, white, and shiny. A wet cast is gray, cool, and has a musty smell. The following rules apply to cast care.

1. Turn the patient as directed by the nurse. All cast surfaces are exposed to the air at one time or another. Even drying is promoted by turning. Do not cover a cast with blankets, plastic, or other material.
2. Use pillows to support the entire length of the cast. When turning and positioning the resident, support the cast with your palms as fingers can make dents in the cast.
3. Protect the resident from rough edges of the cast with tape "petals" or a stockinette.
4. Do not let the resident insert anything into the cast. Sticking objects down the cast can cause skin breakdown.
5. A casted extremity is elevated on pillows. Elevation of an arm or leg reduces swelling.
6. Lying on the injured side is usually not allowed. The nurse instructs the nurse aide as to the appropriate positions.
7. Report pain, swelling, pale skin, cyanosis (blue skin), odor, numbness, temperature changes of skin, inability to move toes and fingers, drainage, chills, or fever.

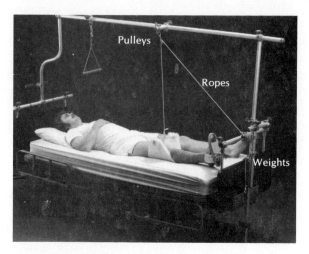

Fig. 9-6. Traction set-up. *(From Perry AG, Potter PA:* Clinical nursing skills and techniques, *ed 2, St Louis, 1990, Mosby–Year Book.)*

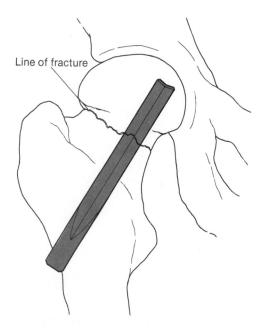

Fig. 9-7 A hip fracture is pinned in place. *(From Miliken ME, Campbell G:* Essential competencies for patient care, *St Louis, 1985, Mosby–Year Book.)*

Traction. Traction may be used to immobilize a fracture. This keeps the fractured bone in place. Weights, ropes, and pulleys are used (Fig. 9-6). Traction can be applied to the neck, arms, legs, or pelvis. Traction is also used for muscle spasms, to correct or prevent deformities, and for other musculoskeletal injuries.

Traction is applied by the doctor to the skin or bone. Skin traction involves applying bandages and strips of material to the skin. Weights are attached to the material or bandage. Traction applied directly to the bone is called skeletal traction. A pin is inserted through the bone, then special devices are attached to the pin. Weights are attached to the device.

Continuous or intermittent traction may be used. Continuous traction is not removed. Intermittent traction can be removed at times ordered by the doctor. Nurse aides should keep the resident in the proper position and pulled up in bed to maintain proper pull. The weights should be kept off the floor. Good skin care is important. Report any signs of breakdown to nurse.

Hip fractures. Fractured hips are common in the elderly. They are especially serious because healing is slower in older people. Other disorders and slow healing may complicate the resident's condition and care. The person is also at great risk for complications following any operation that is needed to correct the fracture.

Open reduction is required. The fracture is fixed in position with a pin (Fig. 9-7). This is called a "hip pinning." A cast or traction is used in some situations and, therefore, care of these patients may also be required. The patient with a hip pinning requires the following care.

1. Give good skin care. Skin breakdown can occur rapidly.
2. Turn and reposition the resident as directed by the nurse. The doctor's orders for turning and positioning depend on the type of fracture and the surgical procedure performed.
3. Keep the operated leg abducted at all times. The legs are abducted (kept apart) when the resident is supine, being turned, or in a side-lying position. Pillows or abductor splints may be used as directed.
4. Prevent external rotation of the hip. Use trochanter rolls or sandbags as directed.
5. Provide a straight-backed chair with armrests or wheelchair when the resident is to be up. A low, soft chair is not used.
6. Place the chair on the unoperated side.
7. Assist the nurse in transferring the resident from a bed to a chair as directed.
8. Do not let the patient stand on the operated leg unless permitted by the doctor.
9. Support and elevate the leg as directed when the resident is in the chair.

Osteoporosis

Osteoporosis is a bone *(osteo)* disorder in which the bone becomes porous and brittle *(porosis)*. It is common in the elderly and women past menopause. A dietary lack of calcium is a major cause of osteoporosis. Bed rest and immobility are other causes because they do not allow for proper bone use. For bone to form properly, it must be used to bear weight. If not, calcium is absorbed and the bone becomes porous and brittle.

Signs and symptoms of osteoporosis include low back pain, gradual loss of height, and stooped posture. Fractures are a major threat. Bones are so brittle that the slightest stress can cause a fracture. Turning in bed or getting up from a chair can cause a fracture. Fractures are a great risk if the resident falls or has an accident.

Osteoporosis is treated with calcium and vitamin supplements. The hormone estrogen may be given to women. Exercise, good posture, and a back brace or corset are also important. Walking aids may be needed. Bed rest is avoided. Caution is used when turning and positioning the resident. The resident must be protected from falls and accidents.

Loss of a limb

An *amputation* is the removal of all or part of an extremity. Usually the part is removed surgically. Amputations are sometimes indicated for severe injuries, bone tumors, severe infections, and circulatory disorders.

Gangrene is a condition in which there is death of tissue. Infection, injuries, and circulatory disorders may result in gangrene. These conditions interefere with blood supply to the tissues. The tissues do not receive enough oxygen and nutrients. Poisonous substances and waste products build up in the affected tissues. Tissue death results. The tissue becomes black, cold, and shriveled (Fig. 9-8), and can eventually fall off. If untreated, gangrene spreads through the body and causes death.

The presence of gangrene may make it necessary for all or part of an extremity to be amputated. Fingers, the hand, forearm, or entire arm may be removed. Toes, the foot, lower leg, upper leg, or entire leg may be amputated. A below-the-knee amputation is called a BK (below the knee) or ABK (amputation below the knee). An above-the-knee amputation is called an AK (above the knee) or AKA (above-the-knee amputation).

After an amputation, the resident needs psychological support. A major psychological adjustment will be necessary. The resident's life will be affected by the amputation. Appearance, activities of daily living, moving about, and job are just a few areas which may be affected.

The resident may be fitted with a prosthesis (Fig. 9-9). The stump must be conditioned for the prosthesis to fit properly. Stump conditioning involves shrinking and shaping the stump into a cone shape. Bandaging is used to shrink and shape the

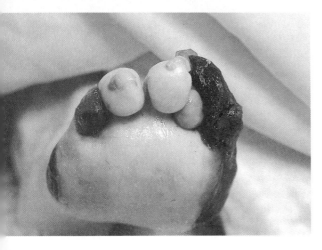

Fig. 9-8 Gangrene.
(From Sorrentino SA: Mosby's textbook for nursing assistants, *ed 3, St Louis, 1992, Mosby–Year Book.)*

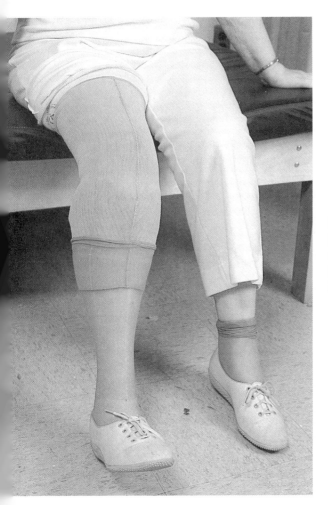

Fig. 9-9 Lower leg prosthesis.
(From Sorrentino SA: Mosby's textbook for nursing assistants, *ed 3, St Louis, 1992, Mosby–Year Book.)*

stump. Exercises are ordered to strengthen the other limbs. Physical therapy helps the resident learn to use the prosthesis. Occupational therapy is necessary if the patient has to learn how to perform activities of daily living with the stump or prosthesis.

The resident may feel that the limb is still there or complain of pain in the amputated part. This is called *phantom limb pain*. The exact cause is unknown. However, it is a normal reaction. The sensation may be present for only a short time after surgery. However, some persons experience phantom limb pain for many years.

CARDIOVASCULAR SYSTEM

Cardiovascular disorders are the leading causes of death in the United States. Problems may occur in the heart or blood vessels. Common examples of cardiovascular disorders are hypertension, coronary artery disease, and congestive heart failure.

Hypertension

Hypertension is a condition in which the blood pressure is too high. Narrowed blood vessels are a common cause of hypertension. When vessels are narrow, the heart has to pump with more force to move blood through the vessels. Kidney disorders, head injuries, some complications of pregnancy, and tumors of the adrenal gland can also cause hypertension.

Hypertension can damage other body organs. The heart may enlarge so it can pump with more force. Blood vessels in the brain may burst and cause a stroke. Blood vessels in the eyes and kidneys may be damaged.

At first, hypertension may not cause signs or symptoms. Usually it is discovered when the blood pressure is measured. Signs and symptoms develop as the disorder progresses. Headache, blurred vision, and dizziness may be reported. Complications of hypertension include stroke, heart attack, kidney failure, and blindness.

Medications to lower the blood pressure may be ordered by the doctor. The resident will be advised to quit smoking, exercise regularly, and get enough rest. A sodium-restricted diet may also be ordered. If the resident is overweight, a low-calorie diet is ordered.

Coronary artery disease

Coronary artery disease (CAD) is a disorder in which the coronary arteries become narrowed. One or all of the arteries may be affected. Because of narrowed vessels, blood supply to the heart muscle is reduced. Atherosclerosis is the most common cause. In atherosclerosis, fatty material collects on the inside of arterial walls.

This causes the arteries to become narrow and obstruct blood flow. Blood flow through an artery may become completely blocked. Permanent heart damage occurs in the part of the heart receiving its blood supply from an artery affected by athero-sclerosis.

Risk factors for the development of CAD include obesity, cigarette smoking, lack of exercise, a diet high in fat and cholesterol, and hypertension. Age and sex are other risk factors. CAD is more common in men and older people. The type A personality is also a risk factor. The person with a type A personality is agressive, competitive, and works very hard. The person has difficulty relaxing, has a sense of urgency, and does things at a rapid pace.

There are two major complications of coronary artery disease. They are angina pectoris and myocardial infarction (heart attack).

Angina pectoris. Angina *(pain)* pectoris *(chest)* means "chest pain." The chest pain is due to reduced blood flow to a part of the heart muscle (myocardium). Angina pectoris is seen when the heart needs additional oxygen. Normally blood flow to the heart increases when the heart's need for oxygen increases. Physical exertion, a heavy meal, emotional stress, and excitement increase the heart's need for oxygen. In CAD the narrowed vessels prevent increased blood flow.

Signs and symptoms of angina pectoris include chest pain. The pain may be described as a tightness or discomfort in the left side of the chest. The pain may radiate to the left jaw, and down the inner side of the left arm. The resident may be pale, feel faint, and perspire. The person may have difficulty breathing. These signs and symptoms cause the patient to stop activity and rest. Rest often relieves the symptoms in 3 to 15 minutes. Rest reduces the heart's need for oxygen. Therefore, normal blood flow is achieved and heart damage is prevented.

Besides rest, angina pectoris is treated with a medication called nitroglycerin. This medication is put under the tongue where it dissolves and is absorbed into the bloodstream.

Residents are taught to avoid situations that are likely to cause angina pectoris. These include overexertion, heavy meals and overeating, and emotional situations. They are advised to stay indoors during cold weather or during hot, humid weather. Exercise programs supervised by doctors may be developed. Some persons need coronary artery bypass surgery. The surgery bypasses the diseased part of the artery and increases blood flow to the heart.

Many residents with untreated angina pectoris eventually have heart attacks. Chest pain that is not relieved by rest and nitroglycerin is probably due to a more serious cause.

Myocardial infarction. A myocardial infarction (MI) is due to lack of blood supply to the heart muscle (myocardium). Tissue death occurs (infarction). Common terms for myocardial infarction are heart attack, coronary, coronary thrombosis, and coronary occlusion. Blood flow to the myocardium is suddenly interrupted. A thrombus usually obstructs blood flow through an artery. The area of damage may be small or large. Cardiac arrest can occur.

Signs and symptoms include sudden, severe chest pain. The pain is usually on the left side. It may be described as crushing, stabbing, or squeezing. Some have described the pain in terms of someone sitting on their chests. The pain may radiate to the neck, jaw, and down the arm. The pain is more severe and lasts longer than angina pectoris. It is not relieved by rest and nitroglycerin. Other symptoms include indigestion, dyspnea, nausea, dizziness, perspiration, pallor, cyanosis (blue skin), cold and clammy skin, low blood pressure, and a weak, irregular pulse. The resident is very fearful and apprehensive. Some have described a feeling of doom. The resident may have all or some of these signs and symptoms.

Myocardial infarction is an emergency. Efforts are directed at relieving the pain, stabilizing vital signs, giving oxygen, and calming the resident. Many medications are given. The resident is treated in a coronary care unit (CCU) which has emergency equipment and drugs. Measures are taken to prevent life-threatening complications. After the resident becomes stable and is transferred out of the CCU, activity is gradually increased. Measures to prevent complications are continued. The resident is discharged back to the facility with specific directions about exercise, activity, medications, and dietary changes.

Congestive heart failure

Congestive heart failure (CHF) occurs when the heart cannot pump blood normally. Blood backs up and causes congestion of tissues. Left-sided heart failure, right-sided heart failure, or both can occur.

When the left side of the heart fails to pump efficiently, blood backs up into the lungs. Signs and symptoms of respiratory congestion occur. These include dyspnea, increased sputum production, cough, and gurgling sounds in the lungs. In addition, blood is not pumped out of the heart to the rest of the body in adequate amounts. Organs receive an inadequate blood supply. Signs and symptoms occur from the body's organs. For example, inadequate blood flow to the brain causes confusion, dizziness, and fainting. Inadequate blood flow to the kidneys causes reduced kidney function and decreased urinary output. The skin becomes pale or cyanotic (blue). Blood pressure falls. Every severe form of left-sided failure is pulmonary edema (fluid in the lungs). Pulmonary edema is an emergency. Death can occur.

The right side of the heart may fail. Blood backs up into the venae cavae and into the venous system. The feet and ankles swell. Neck veins bulge. Congestion occurs in the liver and its function decreases. The abdomen may become congested with fluid. The right side of the heart cannot pump blood to the lungs efficiently. Therefore, normal blood flow does not occur from the lungs to the left side of the heart. Less blood than normal is pumped from the left side of the heart to the rest of the body. Like left-sided failure, the body's organs will have a reduced blood supply. The previously described signs and symptoms then eventually occur.

Congestive heart failure is usually caused by a weakened heart. Myocardial infarction and hypertension are common causes of a weakened heart. Damaged heart valves can also cause CHF.

CHF can be treated and controlled. Drugs are given to strengthen the heart and to reduce the amount of fluid in the body. A sodium-restricted diet is ordered. Supplemental oxygen is given. Most residents prefer semi-Fowler's or Fowler's position for breathing. Many elderly people have CHF. You may be involved in the following aspects of the person's care.

1. Maintaining bed rest or a limited activity program
2. Measuring intake and output
3. Measuring weight daily
4. Restricting fluids as ordered by the doctor
5. Giving good skin care to prevent skin breakdown
6. Performing range-of-motion exercises
7. Assisting with transfers or walking
8. Assisting with self-care activities
9. Maintaining good body alignment
10. Applying elastic stockings

RESPIRATORY SYSTEM

Residents with respiratory disorders are commonly seen in hospitals and nursing facilities. The respiratory system brings oxygen into the lungs and removes carbon dioxide from the body. Respiratory disorders interfere with this function and threaten life. Common respiratory disorders are chronic obstructive pulmonary disease and pneumonia.

Chronic obstructive pulmonary disease

Four disorders are grouped under chronic obstructive pulmonary disease (COPD). They are chronic bronchitis, asthma, bronchiectasis, and emphysema. These disorders interfere with the normal exchange of oxygen and carbon dioxide in the lungs.

Chronic bronchitis. Chronic bronchitis occurs after repeated episodes of bronchitis (inflammation of the bronchial tubes). Common causes are cigarette smoking and air pollution. "Smoker's cough" in the morning is usually the first symptom. At first the cough is dry. Eventually the resident coughs up mucus, which may contain pus and blood. The cough becomes more frequent as the disease progresses. The resident may have difficulty breathing and may tire easily. The mucus and inflamed breathing passages obstruct air flow into the lungs. Therefore, the body cannot get normal amounts of oxygen.

Asthma. Air passages narrow with asthma. Difficulty of breathing results. Allergies and emotional stress are common causes. Episodes occur suddenly and are called asthma attacks. Besides dyspnea, there is shortness of breath, wheezing, coughing, rapid pulse, perspiration, and cyanosis (blue-tinged skin). The person is usually very frightened during the attack. Fear usually causes the attack to become worse.

Drugs are used to treat asthma. Emergency room treatment may be necessary if the attack is severe.

Bronchiectasis. Bronchiectasis is a disorder in which the bronchi dilate (enlarge). Pus collects in the dilated bronchi. There are many causes, including respiratory infections and aspiration. The resident has a chronic, productive cough. Large amounts of sputum are coughed up which contains pus. The sputum usually has a foul smell. The amount increases as the disease progresses. Eventually blood may be present in the sputum. Weight loss, fatigue, and loss of appetite can occur. The doctor may order drugs, respiratory therapy, rest, and measures to improve nutrition. The resident must be protected from others with respiratory infections. Cigarette smoking is not allowed. It may be necessary to remove the diseased part of the lung.

Emphysema. Emphysema is a disorder in which the alveoli (air sacs in the lung) become enlarged. Walls of the alveoli become less elastic. Therefore, they do not expand and shrink normally with inspiration and expiration. As a result, some air is trapped in the alveoli during expiration. The trapped air is not exhaled. As the disease progresses, more alveoli are involved. The normal exchange of oxygen and carbon dioxide cannot occur in the affected alveoli.

Cigarette smoking is the most common cause. Signs and symptoms include shortness of breath and "smoker's cough." At first, shortness of breath occurs with exertion. As the disease progresses, it may occur at rest. Sputum may contain pus. As more air is trapped in the lungs, the patient develops a "barrel chest" (Fig. 9-10). Residents usually prefer to sit upright and slightly forward. Breathing is easier in this position. It's important that the resident stop smoking. Certain medications, breathing treatments, exercises, and oxygen are ordered.

Pneumonia

Pneumonia is an inflammation of lung tissue. The alveoli in the affected area fill with fluid. Because of fluid in the alveoli, oxygen and carbon dioxide cannot be exchanged normally.

Pneumonia is caused by bacteria, viruses, aspiration, or immobility. The resident is very ill. Signs and symptoms include fever, chills, painful cough, pain on breathing, and a rapid pulse. Cyanosis (blue-tinged skin) may be present. The color of sputum produced depends on the cause. Sputum may be clear, green, yellowish, or rusty colored.

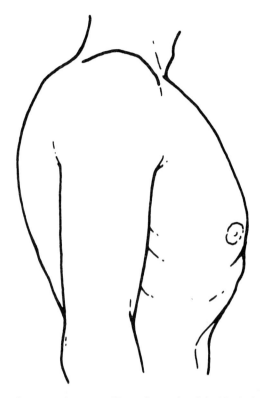

Fig. 9-10 Barrel chest from emphysema. *(From Sorrentino SA:* Mosby's textbook for nursing assistants, *ed 3, St Louis, 1992, Mosby–Year Book.)*

Drugs are ordered for the infection and for pain relief. The doctor may also order "force fluids" because of fever. Fluids also help to thin mucous sections. Thin secretions are easier to cough up. Oxygen may be necessary. Most residents prefer the semi-Fowler's position for breathing. Respiratory isolation may be necessary, depending on the cause. Mouth care is important. Frequent linen changes may be necessary because of fever.

ENDOCRINE SYSTEM

The most common endocrine disorder is diabetes mellitus. In this disorder the body cannot use sugar properly. For proper use of sugar, there must be enough insulin. Insulin is secreted by the pancreas. In diabetes mellitus, the pancreas fails to secrete adequate amounts of insulin. Sugar then builds up in the blood. Cells do not have enough sugar for energy. Therefore, cells cannot perform their specific functions.

Diabetes mellitus occurs in children and adults. Persons at risk are those who have a family history of diabetes. Aging and obesity increase the risk.

Signs and symptoms include increased urine production, increased thirst, hunger, and weight loss. Urine testing shows sugar in the urine. If diabetes is not controlled, complications occur. These include changes in the retina leading to blindness, kidney damage, nerve damage, and circulatory disorders. Circulatory disorders can lead to a stroke, heart attack, and slow healing of wounds. Foot and leg wounds are especially serious. Infection and gangrene often occur and may require amputation of the affected part.

Diabetes mellitus is treated with exercise, diet, and insulin therapy. Meals must be served on time. The resident needs to eat all foods that are served. Urine tests may be ordered. Good foot care is very important.

Insulin shock may develop if a resident gets too much insulin. Diabetic coma develops if a resident does not get enough insulin. Table 4 summarizes the causes, signs, and symptoms of insulin shock and diabetic coma. Both can lead to death if not corrected.

Table 4   Insulin shock and diabetic coma

Insulin shock	Diabetic coma
Causes	
Too much insulin	Undiagnosed diabetes
Omitting a meal	Not enough insulin
Eating an inadequate amount of food	Eating too much food
Excessive physical activity	Insufficient amounts of exercise
Vomiting	Stress from surgery, illness, emotional upset, etc.
Signs and symptoms	
Hunger	Weakness
Weakness	Drowsiness
Trembling	Thirst
Perspiration	Hunger
Headache	Flushed cheeks
Dizziness	Sweet breath odor
Rapid pulse	Slow, deep, and labored respirations
Rapid and weak pulse	Low blood pressure
Low blood pressure	Dry skin
Confusion	Headache
Convulsions	Nausea and vomiting
Cold, clammy skin	Coma
Unconsciousness	

URINARY SYSTEM

During aging, kidney function decreases. There are fewer working units in the kidneys, which can contribute to poisonous substances building up in bloodstream. This can lead to serious health problems. Urine is concentrated because the elderly usually do not drink enough fluids. Urinary frequency also can occur. Bladder retraining programs may be necessary for those with urinary incontinence.

NERVOUS SYSTEM

Nervous system disorders can affect mental and physical functioning. The ability to speak, understand, feel, see, hear, touch, think, control bowels and bladder, or move may be affected. There are many causes and types of nervous system disorders.

Cerebrovascular accident

A cerebrovascular accident (CVA) is commonly called a *stroke*. Blood supply to a part of the brain is suddenly interrupted. Brain damage occurs. The interruption can be due to the rupture of a blood vessel which causes hemorrhage (excessive bleeding) into the brain, or a blood clot can obstruct the blood flow to the brain.

Stroke is more common among the elderly, however persons in their 20s and 30s have had strokes. A common cause of stroke is hypertension (elevated blood pressure). Other risk factors includes diabetes mellitus, obesity, birth control pills, a family history of stroke, hardening of the arteries, smoking, and stress.

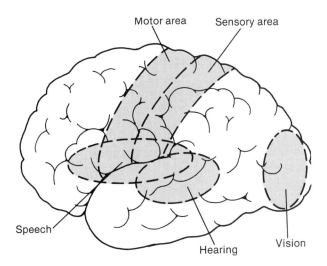

Motor area   Sensory area

Speech

Hearing   Vision

Fig. 9-11 The functions lost from a stroke will depend on the area of brain damage. (*From Miliken ME, Campbell G:* Essential competencies for patient care, *St Louis, 1985, Mosby– Year Book.*)

Signs and symptoms vary. Sometimes there is a warning. The resident may be dizzy, having ringing in the ears, a headache, nausea and vomiting, and memory loss. The stroke may occur suddenly. Unconsciousness, noisy breathing, elevated blood pressure, slow pulse, redness of the face, seizures, and paralysis on one side of the body *(hemiplegia)* may occur. The stroke victim may lose bowel and bladder control and the ability to speak. *Aphasia* is the inability to speak *(phasia)*.

If the person survives, some brain damage is likely. The functions lost depend on the area of brain damaged (Fig. 9-11). Rehabilitation begins immediately. The resident may be partially or totally dependent on others for care. Care of the resident includes:

1. The resident is repositioned frequently (at least every 2 hours) to prevent deformity and aspiration.
2. Coughing and deep breathing are encouraged.
3. Side rails are kept up except when giving care.
4. Elastic stockings (TED hose) are usually ordered to prevent blood clots in the legs.
5. Range-of-motion exercises are performed to prevent contractures.
6. A bladder retraining program is started.
7. A bowel retraining program may be necessary.
8. Safety precautions are practiced.
9. Assistance is given in self-care activities. The resident is encourage to do as much as possible.
10. Methods are established for communicating with the resident. Magic slates, pencil and paper, a picture board, or other methods may be used.
11. Good skin care is given to prevent decubitus ulcers.
12. Speech therapy, physical therapy, and occupational therapy may be ordered.
13. Emotional support and encouragement are given. Praise is given for even the slightest accomplishment.

Parkinson's disease

Parkinson's disease is a slow and progressive disorder. Degeneration of a part of the brain occurs. There is no cure. The disease is usually seen in the elderly. Signs and symptoms are a masklike facial expression, tremors, pill-rolling movements of the fingers, a shuffling gait, stooped posture, stiff muscles, slow movements, slurred speech, monotone speech, and drooling. Mental function is usually not affected early in the disease process. As the disease progresses, confusion and forgetfulness may develop.

Drugs for Parkinson's disease are ordered by the doctor. Physical therapy may also be ordered. The resident may need help eating and with other self-care activities. Measures to promote normal bowel elimination are practiced. There is a risk of constipation because of decreased activity and poor nutrition. Safety practices are carried out to protect the resident from injury. Remember that mental function may not be affected. Treat and talk to the person in an adult manner.

Multiple sclerosis

Multiple sclerosis (MS) is a progressive disease. The myelin sheath (which covers the nerves), the spinal cord, and the white matter in the brain is destroyed. As a result, nerve impulses cannot be sent to and from the brain in a normal manner.

Symptoms begin in young adulthood. The onset is gradual. There is blurred or double vision. Difficulty with balance and walking occur. Tremors, numbness and tingling, weakness, dizziness, urinary incontinence, bowel incontinence or constipation, behavior changes, and incoordination eventually occur. Signs and symptoms progressively worsen over several years. Blindness, contractures, paralysis of all extremities (quadriplegia), loss of bowel and bladder control, and respiratory muscle weakness are among the person's many problems. Eventually the resident becomes totally dependent on others for care.

There is no known cure. Residents are kept active as long as possible. They are encouraged and allowed to do as much for themselves as possible. Nursing care depends on the person's needs and condition. Skin care, personal hygiene, and range-of-motion exercises are important. Residents are protected from injury. Measures are taken to promote bowel and bladder elimination. Turning, positioning, coughing, and deep breathing are also important. Measures are planned to prevent the complications of bedrest.

COMMUNICABLE DISEASES

Communicable (contagious or infectious) diseases can be transmitted from one person to another. They can be transmitted in the following ways.

Direct—from the infected person
Indirect—from dressings, linens, or surfaces
Airborne—from the resident through sneezing or coughing
Vehicle—ingestion of contaminated food, water, drugs, blood, or fluids
Vector—animals, fleas, or ticks

Acquired immunodeficiency syndrome

Acquired immunodeficiency syndrome (AIDS) is caused by a virus. The virus attacks the body's immune system. It affects the person's ability to fight other diseases. There is presently no cure for AIDS and no vaccine to prevent the disease. AIDS eventually causes death. Those at risk for AIDS are:

Homosexual or bisexual men with multiple sex partners
Intravenous drug users
Recent immigrants from Haiti or Central Africa
Sex partners who are homosexual, bisexual, intravenous drug users, or immigrants from Haiti or Central Africa
Children born to infected mothers

AIDS is transmitted mainly by blood or sexual contact. According to the Centers for Disease Control (CDC), the virus that causes AIDS has been found in blood, semen, saliva, tears, urine, vaginal secretions, and breast milk. However, this virus is usually transmitted by contact with infected blood, semen, vaginal secretions, or breast milk.

The virus enters the bloodstream through the rectum, vagina, penis, or mouth. Small breaks in the mucus membrane of the vagina or rectum may occur when the penis, finger, or other objects are inserted. Gum disease can cause breaks in the mucus membrane of the gums. The breaks in the mucus membrane of the mouth, vagina, or rectum provide a route for the virus to enter the bloodstream.

Intravenous drug users transmit AIDS through the use of contaminated needles and syringes. The virus is carried in the contaminated blood left in the needles and syringes. When needles and syringes are used by others, the contaminated blood enters their bloodstreams.

Infection can also occur when infected body fluids come in contact with open areas on the skin. Babies can become infected during pregnancy or shortly after birth.

Some persons infected with the virus that causes AIDS do not develop the disease for many years. They are carriers of the virus. Therefore, they can spread the disease to others.

Some people carry this virus without showing signs or symptoms of the disease. They may not develop the illness for a long time. The signs and symptoms of AIDS include:

Loss of appetite
Weight loss greater than 10 pounds without reason
Fever
Night sweats
Diarrhea
Tiredness (extreme or constant)
Skin rashes
Swollen glands in the neck, underarms, and groin
Dry cough
White spots in the mouth or on the tongue
Purple blotches or bumps on the skin that look like bruises but do not go away

Persons with AIDS develop other diseases. Their bodies do not have the ability to fight disease. The virus that causes AIDS damages the immune system which fights diseases. The person is at risk for pneumonia, Kaposi's sarcoma (a type of cancer), and central nervous system damage. The person with central nervous system damage may show memory loss, loss of coordination, paralysis, and mental disorders.

You may care for persons with AIDS or for persons infected with the virus that causes AIDS. You may have contact with the person's body fluids, or mouth-to-mouth contact is possible during CPR. Certain precautions are necessary to protect yourself and others from AIDS. Universal precautions have been recommended by the CDC. *These precautions apply to all resident contact,* as you may care for a resident who is infected with the virus that causes AIDS but shows no symptoms. It's important that you follow universal precautions at all times.

Hepatitis

Hepatitis is an inflammatory disease of the liver. There are different types of hepatitis.

Type A (infectious hepatitis) is usually spread by the fecal-oral route. Food, water, and drinking or eating containers can be contaminated with feces. The virus is ingested when the person eats or drinks contaminated food or water. It can also be ingested when a person eats or drinks from containers that are contaminated with the virus. Causes include poor sanitation, crowded living conditions, poor nutrition, and poor hygiene practices. You must be careful when handling bedpans, feces, and rectal thermometers. Good handwashing is essential for you and the resident.

Type B (serum hepatitis) is usually transmitted by blood and sexual contact. The type B virus is present in blood, saliva, semen, and urine of infected persons. The virus is spread by contaminated blood or blood products and by sharing needles and syringes among IV drug users.

Hepatitis can be mild in severity or cause death. The signs and symptoms of hepatitis include:

Loss of appetite	Dark urine
Weakness, fatigue, exhaustion	Jaundice (yellowish skin color)
Nausea	Light-colored stools
Vomiting	Headache
Fever	Chills
Skin rash	Abdominal pain

As with AIDS, you must protect yourself and others from the hepatitis virus. Universal precautions are necessary for all health team members.

CANCER

Cancer is a new growth of abnormal cells. The growth is called a *tumor*. Tumors can be benign or malignant (Fig. 9-12). *Benign* tumors grow slowly and within a localized area. They do not usually cause death. *Malignant* tumors grow rapidly and invade other tissues. They cause death if not treated and controlled. The spread of cancer to other parts of the body is called *metastasis*. It occurs if the cancer is not treated and controlled. Cancer can occur in almost any body part. The most common sites are the lungs, colon and rectum, breast, prostate, and uterus.

The exact causes of cancer are unknown. However, certain factors are known to contibute to its development. These include a family history of cancer, exposure to radiation or certain chemicals, smoking, alcohol, food additives, and viruses.

Cancer can be treated and controlled with early detection. The American Cancer Society has identified seven early warning signs of cancer. They are:

1. A change in bowel or bladder habits
2. A sore that does not heal
3. Unusual bleeding or discharge from a body opening
4. A lump or thickening in the breast or elsewhere in the body
5. Difficulty swallowing or indigestion.
6. An obvious change in a wart or mole
7. Nagging cough or hoarseness

The three cancer treatments are surgery, radiotherapy (radiation therapy), and chemotherapy. The treatment depends on the type of tumor, its location, and if it has spread. One or a combination of treatments may be used.

Surgery involves removing malignant tissue. Surgery is done to cure cancer or to relieve pain from advanced cancer. Some surgeries are very disfiguring. These residents have special nursing needs.

Radiotherapy destroys living cells. X-rays are directed at the tumor. Cancer cells and normal cells are exposed to radiation. Both are destroyed. Radiotherapy cures certain cancers, however in some cases it is used only to control the growth of cancer cells. Pain can be relieved or prevented by controlling cell growth. Radiotherapy has side effects. "Radiation sickness" involves discomfort, nausea, and vomiting. Skin breakdown can occur in the exposed area. The doctor may order skin-care procedures.

Chemotherapy involves drugs which kill cells. Like radiotherapy, chemotherapy affects normal cells and cancer cells. It is used to cure cancer or control the rate of cell growth. Side effects can be severe. They are caused by the destruction of normal cells. The gastrointestinal tract is irritated. Nausea, vomiting, and diarrhea result. *Stomatitis*, an inflammation (*itis*) of the mouth (*stomat*), may also develop. Hair loss (alopecia) may occur. Decreased production of blood cells occurs. As a result, the resident is at risk for bleeding and infection. The heart, lungs, liver, kidneys, and skin may also be affected.

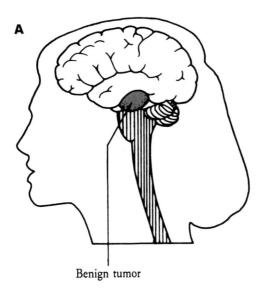

Benign tumor

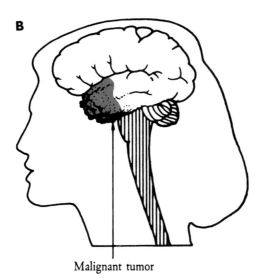

Malignant tumor

Fig. 9-12 A, Benign tumors grow within a localized area. **B,** Malignant tumors invade others. (*From Sorrentino SA:* Mosby's textbook for nursing assistants, *ed 3, St Louis, 1992, Mosby–Year Book.*)

Patients with cancer have many needs. Pain needs to be controlled. Adequate rest and exercise are needed. Fluid and nutritional status must be maintained. Skin breakdown and bowel elimination problems must be prevented. Constipation is a side effect of pain medications. Diarrhea can occur from chemotherapy. The side effects of radiotherapy and chemotherapy must be treated.

The resident's psychological and social needs are great. The person may be angry, afraid, and depressed. Do not avoid the resident because you are uncomfortable. Listen to the resident and use touch to communicate. Being there when your resident needs you is important. You may not have say anything. Just be there to listen.

SUMMARY

A resident may have one or more disorders. For example, a resident may have arthritis, diabetes, heart disease, chronic brain syndrome, and osteoporosis. Problems increase if a fracture occurs. The resident is then at risk for infection, pneumonia, and the complications of bed rest. The amount of care required relates to the nature of the resident's problem and the number of problems. The information in this chapter will help the nurse aide better understand the resident's physical, psychological, and social needs.

Caring for the Resident When Death Is Near

Objectives

Describe terminal illness

Identify two psychological forces that influence living and dying

Describe the five stages of dying

Explain how religion influences attitudes about death

Describe the beliefs about death held by different age groups

Explain how the dying person's psychological, social, and spiritual needs can be met

Explain how you can help meet the physical needs of the dying patient

Describe the needs of the family during the dying process

Describe hospice care

Explain what is meant by a "do not resuscitate" order

Identify the signs of approaching death and the signs of death

Assist in giving postmortem care

Dying people are cared for in hospitals, nursing facilities, or in their homes. Many are part of hospice programs. Death may be sudden and without warning, but often it is expected.

Nurse aides see death often. However, many are unsure of their feelings about death. They are uncomfortable with dying and the subject of death. Sometimes it is seen as a reminder of our eventual deaths.

You must examine your feelings about death. Your attitude about death and dying affects the care you give. You will help meet the resident's physical, psychological, social, and spiritual needs. Therefore, you need to understand the dying process. Then you can approach the dying person with care, kindness, and respect.

TERMINAL ILLNESS

An illness or injury for which there is no reasonable expectation of recovery is a *terminal illness*.

Doctors cannot tell exactly when death will occur from a terminal illness. A person may have days, weeks, months, or years to live. However, predictions have been wrong. People expected to live for only a short time have lived for years. Others that have been expected to live for a longer time died sooner than expected.

Modern medicine has resulted in cures or has prolonged life in many cases. Future research is likely to bring new cures. However, two very powerful psychological forces influence living and dying. They are hope and the will to live. People have died sooner than expected or for no apparent reason when they lost hope or the will to live.

THE STAGES OF DYING

Dr. Elisabeth Kübler-Ross has identified five stages of dying. They are denial, anger, bargaining, depression, and acceptance. During *denial* persons refuse to believe they are dying. "No, not me" is a common response. The person believes a mistake has been made. The person may refuse to listen to information about the illness or injury. The person cannot deal with any problem or decision about the illness or injury. This stage can last for a few hours, days, or much longer. Some people are still in denial when they die.

Anger is the second stage of dying. The person thinks, "Why me?". People in this stage have anger and rage. They envy and resent those who have life and health. Family, friends, and the health team are usually targets of their anger. They blame others. Fault is found with those who are loved and needed the most. The health team and family may have a hard time dealing with residents during this stage. Remember that anger is a normal and healthy reaction. Do not take the person's anger personally. You must control any urge to attack back or avoid the resident.

The third stage is *bargaining*. The anger has passed. The person now says, "Yes, me, but . . ." For example, there is bargaining with God for more time. Promises are made in exchange for more time. The person may want to see a child marry, see a grandchild, have one more Christmas, or live to see some important event. Usually more promises are made as the person makes "just one more" request. This stage may not be obvious to you. Bargaining is usually done privately and on a spiritual level.

Depression is the fourth stage. The person thinks, "Yes, me." The person is very sad. There is mourning over things that have been lost and the future loss of life. The person may cry and say little. Sometimes the person will talk about people and things that will be left behind.

The fifth and final stage of dying is *acceptance* of death. The person is calm and at peace. The person has said what needs to be said. Unfinished business is completed. The person is ready to accept death. A person may be in this stage for many months or years. Reaching acceptance does not mean that death is near.

Dying persons do not always pass through all five stages. A person may never get beyond a certain stage. Or a person may move back and forth between stages. For example, a person who has reached acceptance may move back to bargaining. Then he or she may move forward to acceptance. Some people stay in one stage until death.

ATTITUDES ABOUT DEATH

Experiences, culture, religion, and age influence a person's attitude about death. Many people fear it. Others do not believe they will die. Some look forward to and accept death. Attitudes and beliefs about death often change as a person grows older. They are also affected by changing circumstances.

In the United States, dying people are usually cared for in health facilities. When death occurs, a funeral director is notified. The funeral director takes the body from the facility and prepares it for funeral practices and burial. Consequently, many adults and children have never had contact with a dying person, nor have they been present when death occurred. The process of dying and death is not seen. Therefore it is viewed as mysterious, frightening, and morbid.

These practices and attitudes are different from other cultures where dying people are cared for at home by the family. The family is at the bedside to comfort the dying person and each other. Some families care for the body after death and prepare it for burial.

Attitudes about death are closely related to religion. Some believe that life after death will be free of suffering and hardship. They also believe there will be a reunion with family and loved ones. Many believe there is punishment and suffering for sins and misdeeds in the afterlife. Others do not believe in the afterlife. They believe that death is the end of life. There are also religious beliefs about the form of the human body after death. Some believe that the body keeps its physical form. Others believe that only the spirit keeps its physical form. Another belief is that only the spirit or soul is present in the afterlife. Reincarnation is another belief. *Reincarnation* is the belief that the spirit or soul is reborn into another human body or into another form of life.

Many people strengthen their religious beliefs during the process of dying. Religion is a source of comfort for the dying person and the family. Adults have more fears about death than children. They fear pain and suffering, dying alone, and the invasion of privacy. They also fear loneliness and separation from family and loved ones. They worry about who will care for and support those left behind.

Elderly people usually have fewer fears than younger adults. They are more accepting that death will occur. They have had more experiences with dying and death. Many have lost family members and friends. Some welcome death as freedom from pain, suffering, and disability. However, everyone (young or old) fears dying alone.

PSYCHOLOGICAL, SOCIAL, AND SPIRITUAL NEEDS

Dying people continue to have psychological, social, and spiritual needs. They may want family and friends present. They may want to talk about the fears, worries, and anxieties of dying. Some want to be alone. Often they want to talk to a member of the nursing team. Residents often need to talk during the night. It is quiet and there are few distractions at this time.

There are two important aspects of communication when dealing with the dying resident. These are listening and touch. The resident is the one who needs to talk, express feelings, and share worries or concerns. Just being there and listening helps meet the person's psychological and social needs. Do not worry about saying the wrong thing, nor should you worry about finding the right words to comfort and cheer the person. Nothing really needs to be said. Being there for the resident is what counts. Touch can convey caring and concern when words cannot. Sometimes residents do not want to talk, but need you nearby. Do not feel that you need to talk. Silence, along with touch, is a powerful and meaningful way to communicate.

Spiritual needs are important. The person may wish to see a priest, rabbi, or minister. The person may also want to participate in religious practices. Privacy is provided during spiritual moments. Courtesy is given to the clergy. The resident is allowed to have religious objects nearby such as medals, pictures, statues, or a bible. You must handle these items like other valuables.

PHYSICAL NEEDS

Dying may take a few minutes, hours, days, or weeks. There is a general slowing of body processes, weakness, and changes in the level of consciousness. The resident is allowed to be as independent as possible. As the resident's condition weakens, the nursing team helps meet the resident's basic needs. The resident may totally depend on others for basic needs and activities of daily living. Every effort is made to promote the person's physical and psychological comfort. The person is allowed to die in peace and with dignity.

Vision, hearing, and speech

Vision becomes blurred and gradually fails during the dying process. The resident naturally turns toward light. A darkened room may frighten the resident. The eyes may be half open. Secretions may collect in the corners of the eyes. Because of failing vision, you need to explain what is being done to the resident or in the room. The room should be well lit. However, bright lights and glares are avoided. Good eye care is essential. If the eyes stay open, a nurse may apply a protective ointment. Then the eyes are covered with moistened pads to protect them from injury.

Speech becomes difficult. It may be hard to understand the resident. Sometimes the person cannot speak. The nursing team needs to anticipate the resident's needs. "Yes" or "no" questions are asked. These are kept to a minimum. Though speech may be hard or impossible for the resident, you must still talk to him or her.

Hearing is one of the last functions to be lost during the dying process. Many people hear until the moment of death. Even if unconscious, the person may hear. Always assume that the dying person, or any unconscious resident, can hear. Speak in a normal voice, provide reassurance and explanations about care, and offer words of comfort. Topics that could upset the patient are avoided.

Mouth, nose, and skin

Oral hygiene is important for comfort. Routine mouth care is usually adequate if the resident can eat and drink. Frequent oral hygiene is given as death approaches and when there is difficulty taking oral fluids. Oral hygiene is also important if mucus collects in the mouth and the resident cannot swallow.

Crusting and irritation of the nostrils can occur. Common causes are increased nasal secretions, an oxygen cannula, or an NG tube. Careful cleansing of the nose is important. The nurse may have you apply a lubricant to the nostrils.

Circulation fails and body temperature rises as death approaches. The skin is cool and pale. Perspiration increases. Good skin care, bathing, and the prevention of sores are necessary. Linens and gowns are changed as often as needed. Although the skin feels cool, only light bed coverings may be needed. Blankets may make the person feel too warm and cause restlessness.

Elimination

Persons who are dying may have urinary and anal incontinence. Waterproof bed protectors are used. Perineal care is given as necessary. Some residents are constipated and have urinary retention. Doctors may order enemas. Foley catheters may be ordered for urinary retention or incontinence. You may be responsible for giving enemas and catheter care.

Comfort and positioning

Measures are taken to promote comfort. Good skin care, personal hygiene, back massages, and oral hygiene help to increase comfort. Some residents have severe pain. They need strong pain medications which are given by nurses. You can also promote comfort by frequent position changes. Good body alignment using support also promotes comfort. The resident should be turned carefully. Residents with breathing difficulties usually prefer the semi-Fowler's position.

The resident's room

The resident's room should be as pleasant as possible. The room should be well ventilated and well lit. Unnecessary equipment is removed. The resident should be watched carefully, so the dying resident is often placed in a room close to the nurse's station.

Momentos, pictures, cards, flowers, religious objects, and other significant items comfort and reassure the resident. Arranging them within the resident's view is appreciated. The resident and family is allowed to arrange the room according to the resident's wishes. This helps meet the needs of love, belonging, and esteem. The room should be comfortable, pleasant, and reflect the person's choices. This promotes physical and psychological comfort.

NEEDS OF THE RESIDENT'S FAMILY

The family is going through a hard time. It may be very hard to find the right words to comfort them. You can show your feelings to the family by being available, courteous, and considerate. Also use touch to show your concern.

The family is usually allowed to spend a lot of time with their loved one. Normal visiting hours usually do not apply if the resident is dying. You must respect the resident's and family's right to privacy. They need as much time together as possible. However, resident care cannot be neglected just because the family is present. Most facilities let family members help give care if they wish to do so. If they do not want to help, you can suggest that they take a break. They can use the time to have a beverage or meal.

The family may be tired, sad, and tearful. They need support and understanding. Watching a loved one die is painful, and so is dealing with the eventual loss of that person. The family must be given every possible courtesy and respect. They may find comfort in a visit from a member of the clergy. Communicate this request to the nurse immediately.

HOSPICE CARE

Some residents and families seek hospice care. Hospices are concerned with the physical, emotional, social, and spiritual needs of dying residents and their families. Hospices are not concerned with cures or life-saving procedures. Rather, they emphasize pain relief and comfort measures. The goal of hospice care is to improve the dying person's quality of life.

A hospice may be part of a health-care facility or a separate facility. Many hospices offer home care. Follow-up care and support groups for survivors are also part of hospice services.

"DO NOT RESUSCITATE" ORDERS

When death is sudden and unexpected, every effort is made to save the person's life. CPR is started and an emergency ' ode" is called. CPR and other life support measures are continued until the person is resuscitated or until the resident is declared dead by a doctor.

Doctors often write "do not resuscitate" (DNR) or "no code" orders for terminal residents. This means that no attempts will be made to resuscitate the person. The person will be allowed to die in peace and with dignity. The orders are often written after the resident or family has been consulted. Some residents have written instructions about life-prolonging measures. These are called "living wills." A living will usually states that the person does not want his or her life prolonged by extraordinary means if there is no reasonable expectation of recovery.

SIGNS OF DEATH

You need to know the signs of approaching death. These signs may occur rapidly or gradually.

1. Movement, muscle tone, and sensation are lost. This usually begins in the feet and legs. It eventually spreads to the rest of the body. When the mouth muscles relax, the jaw drops. The mouth may stay open. There is often a peaceful facial expression.
2. Peristalsis and other gastrointestinal functions slow down. There may be abdominal distention, anal incontinence, impaction, nausea, and vomiting.
3. Circulation fails and body temperature rises. The person feels cool or cold, looks pale, and perspires heavily. The pulse is fast, weak, and irregular. The blood pressure begins to fall.
4. As the respiratory system fails, Cheyne-Stokes, slow, or rapid and shallow respirations may be observed. Mucus accumulates in the respiratory tract. This causes the "death rattle" to be heard.
5. Pain decreases as the resident loses consciousness. However, some people are conscious until the moment of death.

The signs of death include no pulse, respirations, or blood pressure. The pupils are fixed and dilated. A doctor determines that death has occurred and pronounces the person dead.

CARE OF THE BODY AFTER DEATH

Care of the body after *(post)* death *(mortem)* is called *postmortem* care. A nurse is responsible for postmortem care. You may be asked to assist. The care begins as soon as the doctor pronounces the patient dead. Universal precautions are followed when giving postmortem care since the patient may have infected body fluids or body substances.

Postmortem care is done to maintain good appearance of the body. Discoloration and skin damage are prevented. Postmortem care also includes gathering valuables and personal possessions for the family. The right to privacy and the right to be treated with dignity and respect also apply after death.

Within 2 to 4 hours after death, rigor mortis develops. *Rigor mortis* is the stiffness or rigidity *(rigor)* of skeletal muscles after death *(mortis)*. Postmortem care involves positioning the body in normal alignment before rigor mortis sets in. There is another reason for placing the body in a normal position. The family may wish to see the body before it is taken to the morgue or funeral home. The body should appear in a comfortable and natural position for viewing.

POSTMORTEM CARE

To assist with postmortem care, gather the following equipment: postmortem kit, valuable list, bed protector, wash basin, washcloth, towels, dressing, and gloves. Apply the gloves and place the body in the supine position. Gently close the eyes and apply a moistened cotton ball over each eyelid. Insert dentures if it is facility policy.

Close the resident's mouth. Place a towel roll under the chin if the mouth will not stay in a closed position. Remove jewelry except for wedding rings. List jewelry on the valuable list and place in an envelope. Some facilities require that this be witnessed. The envelope should be given to the family. Remove drainage bottles, bags, and containers. Leave tubes and catheters in place if an autopsy is to be performed. If you have any questions, ask the charge nurse.

Bathe and dry the body. Place a bed protector under the buttocks. Replace soiled dressings. Put a clean gown on the body. Brush and comb the hair. Fill out identification tags and attach to the body. After the family views the body, the shroud is applied. Transport the body to the morgue.

SUMMARY

Many people die in health facilities. Therefore, health workers see death often. You may be uncomfortable with the subject of death. If so, you will be uncomfortable with dying. Some people feel that medicine should be able to keep people alive longer. These people will be angry and frustrated with the dying resident. Certain behaviors are seen when health workers do not feel comfortable with death and dying. These include avoiding the resident, nervous talking, hurried care, rough handling, and reducing the importance of a resident's needs. You may need to discuss your feelings about death with a nurse, other health workers, or a member of the clergy. This will help you develop a more positive attitude about death.

The terminally ill resident should be allowed to die with peace and dignity. The person is encouraged to be independent for as long as possible. As the person's condition weakens, the nursing team is needed more and more for care and comfort. Even though the person is dying, basic needs continue.

The health team is concerned with the dying person's psychological, social, and spiritual comfort. Visits from the clergy are often appreciated by the resident.

The nurse aide uses various ways to communicate with the dying resident, including silence and touch. Privacy must be respected before and after death.

Postmortem care is given after death. Each facility has policies and procedures about caring for the body after death. The resident's body is treated with dignity and respect.

CHAPTER 11

Bathing, Grooming, and Dressing

Objectives

Explain the importance of cleanliness and skin care

Describe the routine resident care performed before and after breakfast, after lunch, and in the evening

Describe the general rules related to bathing residents and the observations to make

Identify the safety precautions for residents taking tub baths or showers

Identify the purposes of perineal care

Explain the importance of oral hygiene and list the observations to report

Identify the purposes of a back massage

Explain the importance of hair care and shaving

Explain the importance of nail and foot care

Cleanliness and skin care are necessary for comfort, safety, and health. The skin is the body's first defense against disease. Intact skin prevents microorganisms from entering the body and causing an infection. Likewise, mucous membranes of the mouth, genital area, and anus must be kept clean and intact. Besides cleansing, hygiene practices prevent body and breath odors, promote relaxation, and increase circulation.

Culture and personal choice influence hygiene. Some people like to shower. Others like tub baths. One person may bathe at bedtime. Another may bathe in the morning. The frequency of bathing also varies among individuals.

Residents usually need help with personal hygiene. Weakness due to illness and bodily changes from aging affect the ability to practice hygiene. The need for cleanliness and skin care is affected by perspiration, vomiting, urinary and bowel elimination, drainage from wounds or body openings, bedrest, and activity. The charge nurse decides the amount and type of personal hygiene you need to provide for an individual.

DAILY CARE OF THE RESIDENT

Personal hygiene is performed as often as necessary to stay clean and comfortable. Teeth are brushed and face and hands washed after rising in the morning. These and other hygiene measures may be done routinely before meals, after meals, and at bedtime.

Before breakfast

Routine care before breakfast is often called *early morning care* or *AM care*. The night shift or day shift staff may be responsible for AM care. They get residents ready for breakfast. Personal hygiene measures performed at this time include:

1. Toileting residents.
2. Helping residents wash their faces and hands.
3. Assisting residents with oral hygiene.
4. Assisting residents with dressing.
5. Positioning residents in the Fowler's position in bed.
6. Straightening or changing bed linens.
7. Straightening the residents' room.

After breakfast

Morning care is given after breakfast. Routine morning care usually involves providing showers, tub baths, or bedbaths and assisting with oral hygiene, shaving, hair care, toileting, and dressing.

Evening care

Care given at bedtime is called *HS care*. Hygiene measures are performed right before the resident is ready for sleep. They help promote comfort and relaxation. HS care involves:

1. Toileting residents.
2. Helping residents wash their faces and hands.
3. Assisting residents with oral hygiene.
4. Changing damp or soiled linens and straightening all other linens.
5. Assisting residents in putting on gowns or pajamas.
6. Giving back massages.
7. Straightening the residents' room.

BATHING

Besides cleansing, bathing has other purposes. A bath is refreshing and relaxing. Circulation is stimulated and body parts exercised. Observations can be made during the bath.

A resident may get a complete or partial bed bath, a tub bath, or a shower. The method depends on the resident's condition, ability to provide self-care, and personal choice. In health facilities, bathing usually occurs after breakfast. Again, personal choice needs to be considered regarding time of day and frequency. A person who bathes at bedtime should be allowed to continue the practice if possible.

The frequency of bathing is an individual matter. Some people bathe at least once a day. Others take a complete bath only once or twice a week. Personal choice, the weather, physical activity, and illness influence how often a person bathes. Illness usually increases the need for bathing because of fever and increased perspiration. Other illnesses and dry skin may require bathing every 2 or 3 days.

Skin-care products

There are many kinds of skin-care products. Some are used for cleansing. Others protect the skin from drying or friction. The products used depend on personal choice and cost.

Soaps cleanse the skin. They remove dirt, dead skin, skin oil, some microorganisms, and perspiration. However, they tend to dry and irritate the skin. Dry skin is easily injured and causes itching and discomfort. Skin must be rinsed well to remove all soap.

Soap is not needed for every bath. Plain water can clean the skin. Plain water is often used for the elderly because of their dry skin. People with dry skin may prefer soaps containing bath oils. Soaps should not be used if a person has very dry skin.

Bath oils keep the skin soft and prevent drying. Some soaps contain bath oils, or liquid bath oil can be added to bath water. Showers and tubs become slippery from bath oils. Safety precautions are needed to prevent falls.

Creams and lotions protect skin from the drying effect of air and evaporation. They do not feel greasy but leave an oily film on the skin. Most are scented.

Powders absorb moisture and prevent friction when two skin surfaces rub together. They are usually applied under the breasts, under the arms, and in the groin area. Sometimes powders are applied between the toes. Powder is applied to dry skin in a thin, even layer. Excessive amounts of powder cause caking and crusts that can cause skin irritation.

Deodorants and antiperspirants are applied to the axillae (underarms) after bathing. *Deodorants* mask and control body odors. *Antiperspirants* reduce the amount of perspiration. Deodorants and antiperspirants should not be applied to irritated skin.

Observations

When bathing a resident or when assisting a resident to bathe, you should observe the skin. The following observations are reported to the nurse.

1. The color of the skin, lips, nail beds, and sclera (whites of the eyes)
2. The location and description of rashes

3. Dry skin
4. Bruises or open areas of the skin
5. Pale or reddened areas, particularly over bony parts
6. Drainage or bleeding from wounds or body openings
7. Skin temperature
8. Resident complaints of pain or discomfort

General rules

Certain rules must be followed for bed baths, showers, or tub baths. They are:

1. Ask the nurse what type of bath a resident is to have. Find out which skin care products to use. The resident's personal choice should be allowed when possible.
2. Collect necessary equipment before beginning the procedure, including bed linen.
3. Protect the resident's privacy. Properly screen the resident and close doors.
4. Make sure the resident is adequately covered for warmth and privacy.
5. Reduce drafts by closing doors and windows.
6. Protect the resident from falling, keep the opposite side rail up at all times.
7. Use good body mechanics at all times.
8. Make sure the water is at the proper temperature (110° to 115° F for bed bath). Change the water often throughout the procedure.
9. Keep soap in the soap dish between latherings. This prevents the water from becoming real soapy. If a tub bath is taken, the resident will not slip on the soap.
10. Wash from the cleanest to the dirtiest areas, wash and dry one body part at a time, head to toe.
11. Encourage the resident to help as much as possible. Promote safety measures.
12. Rinse the skin thoroughly to remove all soap.
13. Pat the skin dry to avoid irritating or breaking the skin.
14. Bathe the skin whenever fecal material or urine is on the skin.

Complete bed bath

The *complete bed bath* involves washing the resident's entire body in bed. Residents who are unconscious, paralyzed, in a cast or traction, or weak from illness or surgery generally require bed baths. Complete bed baths are given to residents who cannot bathe themselves.

Ask the nurse about the resident's ability to assist in the bath. Also ask about any limitations in activity or position. Consult with the nurse about the need for universal precautions.

During the bed bath, keep the resident covered to protect privacy. Provide explanation of procedures.

Partial bath

The partial bath involves bathing the face, hands, axillae (underarms), genital area, back, and buttocks. These body areas may develop odors or cause discomfort if they are not clean. Partial bed baths are given to residents who cannot help themselves and to residents on opposite days of their scheduled baths or showers. Residents who are able can bathe themselves in bed or at the bathroom sink. Nursing personnel assists as needed, especially in washing the back.

The general rules for bathing apply for partial bed baths. The considerations involved in giving a complete bed bath also apply.

Tub bath

Many people like tub baths. Residents may find them relaxing. They must be protected from falling when getting in and out of tubs and from burns due to hot water (water temperature should be 105° F). A tub bath can cause a person to feel faint, weak, or tired. These are more likely to occur if the person has been prescribed bed rest. A bath should not last longer than 20 minutes.

Do not let a resident take a tub bath unless the nurse gives approval. Some residents have private baths. If not, you need to make sure the tub room is available. The tub should be cleaned before being used. A bath mat must be on the bottom of the tub to help prevent falls.

For safety, you may want to drain the tub before the resident gets out. If the tub is drained first, keep the resident covered and protected from exposure and chilling. Changes in the procedure may be necessary for some residents. Consult with the nurse before assisting a resident with a tub bath.

Shower

A shower may be part of the bathtub design or a separate stall. A shower stall has advantages. The resident can walk into the stall rather than having to step over the side of the tub. Weak and paralyzed residents can use a shower chair which is wheeled into the shower stall. Shower chairs are made of plastic with wheels on the legs. A round, open area in the seat lets water drain (Fig. 11-1). The chair can be used to transport the person to and from the shower room. The wheels must be locked during the shower to prevent the chair from moving. A straight-backed chair or a stool can be used if a shower chair is not available.

Residents must be protected from falling and chilling. Their privacy must also be protected. Weak or unsteady residents are not allowed to stand in the shower. They are not left unattended. Encourage residents to use the hand rails for support when getting in and out of the shower. Hand rails are especially important if the shower is in tub.

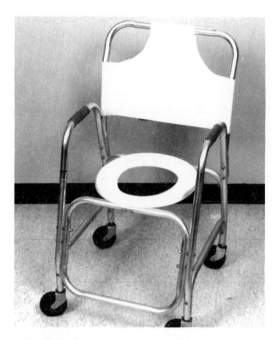

Fig. 11-1 A shower chair. *(From Sorrentino SA:* Mosby's textbook for nursing assistants, *ed 3, St Louis, 1992, Mosby–Year Book.)*

PERINEAL CARE

Perineal care (pericare) involves cleaning the genital and anal areas. These areas are warm, moist, and dark. They provide a place for microorganisms to grow. The genital and anal areas are cleaned to prevent infection and odors and to promote comfort.

Perineal care is done at least once a day and is included as part of the bath procedure on bath days. The procedure is also done whenever the area is contaminated with urine or feces. Residents with certain disorders need perineal care more often.

Residents should do their own perineal care if able. Otherwise it is given by nursing personnel. Residents may not know the terms perineum and perineal. Most people understand one or more of the following terms "privates," "private parts," "crotch," "genitals," or "the area between your legs." Be sure to use a term that the resident understands. The term should also be in good taste professionally.

Universal precautions and the rules of medical asepsis are followed. You will work from the cleanest area to the dirtiest. The urethral area is the cleanest and the anal area is the dirtiest. The perineal area is delicate and easily injured. When washing the female resident, separate the labia. When washing the male, retract the foreskin if he is uncircumcised to clean the penis. Warm water, not hot is used. The area must be rinsed thoroughly. The perineum is patted dry after rinsing to reduce moisture and promote comfort. Protect the resident's privacy by covering the resident and pulling the screen.

ORAL HYGIENE

Oral hygiene, or mouth care, keeps the mouth and teeth clean. A clean mouth and clean teeth prevent mouth odors and infections, increase comfort, and make food taste better. Illness and disease may cause the resident to have a bad taste in the mouth. Some drugs and diseases cause the mouth and tongue to be coated with a whitish material. Other drugs and diseases cause redness and swelling of the mouth and tongue.

The nurse decides the type of mouth care and amount of assistance an individual needs. Oral hygiene is provided upon awakening, after meals, and at bedtime. Many people also practice oral hygiene before meals.

Equipment

A toothbrush, toothpaste, dental floss, and mouthwash are needed. The toothbrush should have soft or medium bristles. Residents with dentures need a denture cleaner, a denture cup, and a denture brush or regular toothbrush. Toothettes are used for residents with sore and tender mouths and for unconscious or comatose residents. A *toothette* is a piece of spongy foam attached to a stick. Other needed items include an emesis basin, water glass, straw, tissues, and towels.

Many people bring their oral hygiene equipment from home. The nursing facility may also provide oral hygiene materials.

Universal precautions are necessary when giving oral hygiene. You will have contact with the person's mucous membranes. Gums may bleed during oral care. Also, many pathogens are in the mouth. Pathogens spread through sexual contact may be in the mouths of some individuals.

Brushing teeth

The amount of assistance needed for toothbrushing varies. Many people perform oral hygiene themselves. Others need help in gathering and setting up the equipment. You may have to brush the teeth of residents who are weak or unable to use or move their arms. The following are reported to the nurse if observed when teeth are brushed.

1. Dry, cracked, swollen, or blistered lips
2. Redness, swelling, irritation, sores, or white patches in the mouth or on the tongue
3. Bleeding, swelling, or redness of the gums

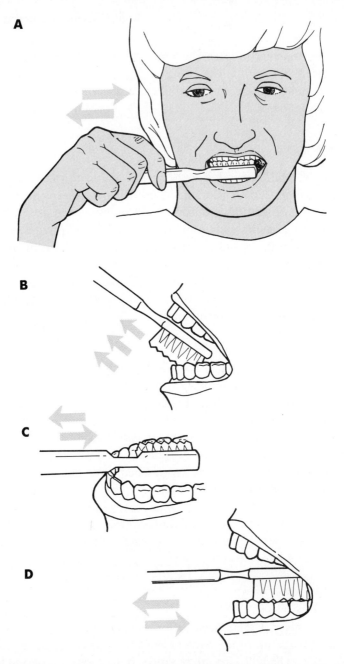

Fig. 11-2 A, Position toothbrush horizontally and brush back and forth with short strokes. **B,** Position brush at a 45° angle against inside of front teeth. Brush from gum to crown of tooth with short strokes. **C,** Hold brush horizontally against the inner surfaces of teeth and brush back and forth. **D,** Position the brush on the biting surfaces of the teeth and brush back and forth. *(From Sorrentino SA:* Mosby's textbook for nursing assistants, *ed 3, St Louis, 1992, Mosby–Year Book.)*

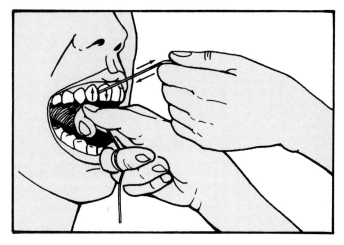

Fig. 11-3 Flossing teeth. *(From Sorrentino SA:* Mosby's textbook for nursing assistants, *ed 3, St Louis, 1992, Mosby–Year Book.)*

To assist a resident in brushing the teeth, the nurse aide can bring equipment to bedside and set it up on the overbed table or can set the equipment up at the lavoratory. Have a resident brush the teeth gently (Fig. 11-2) and rinse thoroughly with water or diluted mouthwash.

Flossing

Flossing removes plaque and tarter from teeth. These substances can cause serious gum disease, resulting in loosening and loss of teeth. Therefore, dental flossing is a preventive measure. Flossing is also done to remove food between the teeth. Flossing is usually done after brushing but can be done at other times. Some people floss after meals. If only done once a day, bedtime is the best time to floss.

There is waxed and unwaxed dental floss. Waxed floss does not fray as easily as the unwaxed type. Some people find waxed floss easier to use because it slides between the teeth. However, particles on tooth surfaces are more likely to attach to unwaxed floss. Many dentists recommend unwaxed floss, which is thinner than waxed floss.

You need to floss for the resident if he or she cannot tend to oral hygiene (Fig. 11-3).

Mouth care for the unconscious or comatose resident

Unconscious residents need special mouth care. They cannot eat and drink, they breathe with their mouths open, and are usually receiving supplemental oxygen. These factors cause mouths to become dry and crusts to form on tongues and mu-

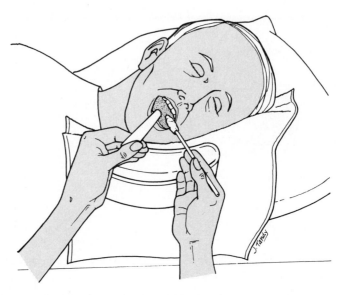

Fig. 11-4 The head of the unconscious or comatose resident is turned well to the side to prevent the possibility of aspiration. The nurse aide uses a padded tongue blade to keep the mouth open while cleaning with applicators. *(From Sorrentino SA:* Mosby's textbook for nursing assistants, *ed 3, St Louis, 1992, Mosby–Year Book.)*

cous membranes. Good mouth care keeps the mouth clean and moist and helps prevent infection.

Lemon glycerine swabs are often used to give mouth care to these residents. However, they have a drying effect and should not be the only method of mouth care used. Toothettes dipped in a small amount of mouthwash, hydrogen peroxide, or a salt solution can be used to clean the mouth. Petroleum jelly or other lubricant is applied to the lips after cleaning to prevent them from cracking.

Unconscious residents usually cannot swallow and must be protected from choking and aspiration. *Aspiration* is the breathing of fluid into the lungs. To prevent aspiration, position the resident on one side with the head turned well to the side with a towel under the head (Fig. 11-4). This position allows excess fluid to run out of the mouth, reducing the risk of aspiration. Using only a small amount of fluid also helps reduce the possibility of aspiration.

The resident's mouth must be kept open for mouth care. A padded tongue blade can be used for this. A padded tongue blade is made by placing two tongue blades together, wrapping gauze around the top half, and taping the gauze into place. Do not hold the mouth open with your fingers. The resident can bite down on them. Microorganisms can enter your body through the broken skin and cause an infection. Universal precautions should be followed.

Unconscious residents cannot speak or respond to what is happening. However, always assume they can hear. Explain what you are doing step by step. Also tell the resident when you are finished and when you are leaving the room.

Mouth care may be needed every 2 hours. Check with the charge nurse and the nursing care plan to see how often it is to be done and the solution to be used. These residents should also be repositioned every 2 hours. Combining mouth care, skin care, and other comfort measures increases their comfort and safety.

Denture care

Dentures are cleaned for persons who cannot do so themselves. Mouth care is provided and dentures cleaned as often as natural teeth. Remember that dentures are the person's property and they are expensive. Losing or damaging dentures is negligent conduct.

Dentures are slippery when wet. They are held firmly over a basin of water lined with a towel when being cleaned. They can easily break or chip if dropped onto a hard surface. Hot water causes them to warp. Do not use hot water to clean or store dentures. Some residents do not wear their dentures. If not worn, they are stored in a container of cool water. Dentures can dry out and warp if not stored in water.

To provide denture care, assist the resident in removing them by grasping the denture with the thumb and index finger (Fig. 11-5). Use universal precautions when providing denture care. Brush the dentures using a back and forth motion to

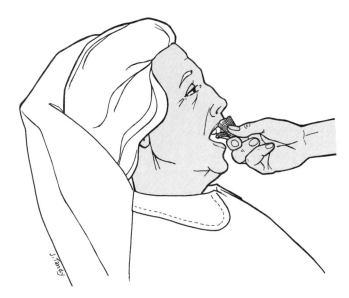

Fig. 11-5 Removing dentures. *(From Sorrentino SA:* Mosby's textbook for nursing assistants, *ed 3, St Louis, 1992, Mosby–Year Book.)*

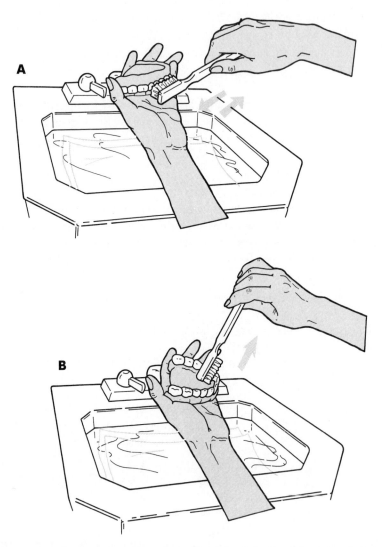

Fig. 11-6 A and **B,** Cleansing dentures. (*From Sorrentino SA:* Mosby's textbook for nursing assistants, *ed 3, St Louis, 1992, Mosby–Year Book.*)

clean the front and vertical brush motions to clean the inner surfaces. Rinse the dentures thoroughly and assist the resident in inserting the dentures. The resident should rinse with water or diluted mouthwash to remove any food particles and to freshen breath prior to reinserting the dentures (Fig. 11-6).

THE BACK MASSAGE

The back massage, or back rub, relaxes muscles and stimulates circulation. The massage is normally given after the bath and as a part of HS care. It should last 4 to 6 minutes. Observe the skin for abnormalities before beginning.

Lotion is used to reduce friction when giving the massage. It should be warmed before being applied. Place the lotion bottle in the bath water or hold it under warm running water to warm. Another way to warm lotion is to rub some between your hands.

The prone position is best for a massage. The side-lying position is often used. Firm strokes are used and your hands should always be in contact with the resident's skin (Fig. 11-7). Always provide for privacy when giving a back massage.

Back rubs may not be given to all residents. They may be dangerous for those with certain heart diseases, back injuries, back surgeries, skin diseases, and some lung disorders. Check with the nurse before giving back massages to residents with these disorders.

HAIR CARE

Appearance and mental well-being are affected by how the hair looks and feels. Illness and disability may prevent people from doing hair care. Residents are assisted with hair care whenever necessary. Some facilities have barbers and beauticians for cutting, shampooing, and styling hair.

Brushing and combing hair

Brushing and combing are part of morning care. They are also done at other times of the day if needed. Many people like to have their hair styled before visitors arrive. Encourage residents to do their own hair care. However, provide assistance as needed. Hair care is done for those who cannot do so. Let the resident choose how the hair is to be brushed, combed, and styled.

Long hair is easily matted and tangled when lying in bed. Daily brushing and combing helps prevent this problem. Braiding also prevents matting and tangling (Fig. 11-8). Do not braid hair unless the resident gives permission. Never cut hair to remove mats or tangles.

When giving hair care, protect the resident's gown or clothing by placing a towel across the shoulders. If hair care is provided with the resident in bed, it is done be-

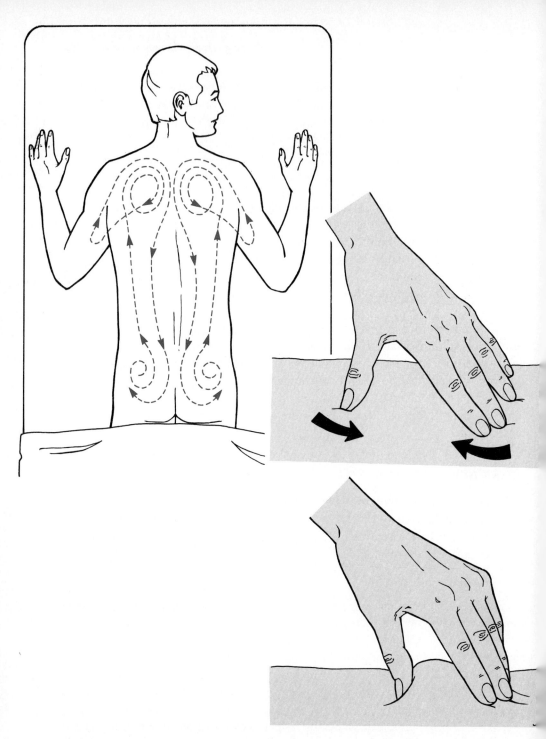

Fig. 11-7 Resident lies in prone position for a back massage. The nurse aide strokes upward from the buttocks to the shoulders, down over the upper arms, back up the upper arms, across the shoulders, and down the back to the buttocks. *(From Sorrentino SA:* Mosby's textbook for nursing assistants, *ed 3, St Louis, 1992, Mosby–Year Book.)*

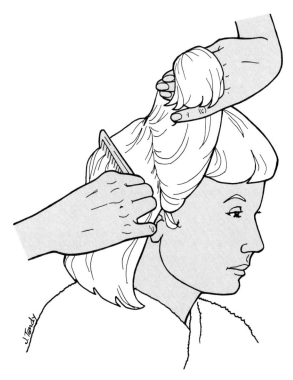

Fig. 11-8 Resident's hair being combed. *(From Sorrentino SA:* Mosby's textbook for nursing assistants, *ed 3, St Louis, 1992, Mosby–Year Book.)*

fore changing the pillowcase. If done after a linen change, place a towel across the pillow to collect falling hair. Always provide for the resident's privacy and safety.

Shampooing

Most people wash their hair at least once a week. Some shampoo two or three times a week. Others shampoo every day. Many factors influence how often shampooing is done. These include the condition of the hair and scalp, hair style, and personal choice. Shampoo and hair conditioner also are determined by personal choice.

Residents in a nursing facility probably need help shampooing. Personal choice is followed whenever possible. However, safety is necessary and the nurse's approval is needed.

There are several ways to shampoo hair. The method used depends on the person's condition, safety, and personal choice if possible. The nurse decides which method to use. Hair is dried and styled as quickly as possible after shampooing. Women may want their hair curled or rolled up before drying. Consult with the nurse before curling or rolling up hair.

Shampooing during the shower or tub bath. Residents who can shower will probably be able to shampoo at the same time. Shampooing can also be done for those using shower chairs. A hand-held shower nozzle is used. It can also be used during a tub bath. A spray of water is directed to the hair. Make sure the water is at the proper temperature. Provide for safety and privacy. The person shampooing during a tub bath will probably need help. An extra towel, shampoo, and hair conditioner (if requested) should be within the person's reach.

A shampoo at the sink. An individual who can sit in a chair can usually be shampooed at a sink. The chair is placed so the person faces away from the sink. The person's head is tilted back over the edge of the sink. A folded towel is placed over the sink edge to protect the neck. A water pitcher or hand-held nozzle is used to wet and rinse the hair.

A shampoo in bed. A shampoo can be given in bed. This method is used for those who cannot sit in a chair. A rubber or plastic trough is placed under the head to protect the linens and mattress from water. The trough also drains water into a basin placed on a chair by the bed (Fig. 11-9). A water pitcher is used to wet and rinse the hair. The water should be about 110° F. Protect the resident's eyes. Provide for privacy.

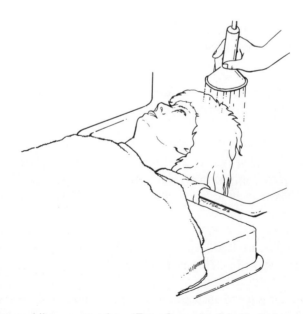

Fig. 11-9 Shampoo while on a stretcher. (*From Sorrentino SA:* Mosby's textbook for nursing assistants, *ed 3, St Louis, 1992, Mosby–Year Book.*)

SHAVING

A shaven face is important for the comfort and well-being of many men. Likewise, most women shave their legs and underarms. Residents may prefer electric shavers or razor blades. When using an electric shaver, practice safety precautions for using electrical equipment. Razor blades can cause nicks or cuts. Universal precautions may be necessary to prevent contact with the resident's blood.

The beard and skin are softened before shaving with a razor blade. The skin is softened by applying a warm washcloth or face towel to the face for a few minutes. Then the face is lathered with soap and water or a shaving cream (Fig. 11-10). Be careful not to cut or irritate the skin while shaving. Women's legs and underarms can be shaved after the bath when the skin is soft. Soap and water or a shaving cream can also provide a lather for shaving the legs and underarms.

Many men have beards and mustaches, which need daily grooming. Ask the resident how he prefers to have them groomed.

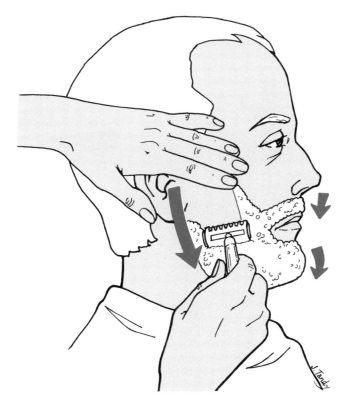

Fig. 11-10 Shaving is done in the direction of hair growth. (*From Sorrentino SA:* Mosby's textbook for nursing assistants, *ed 3, St Louis, 1992, Mosby–Year Book.*)

CARE OF NAILS AND FEET

Nails and feet need special attention to prevent infection, injury, and odors. Hangnails, ingrown nails (nails that grow in at the side), and nails torn away from the skin cause breaks in the skin. These breaks let microorganisms enter the body. Long or broken nails can scratch the skin or snag clothing. Dirty feet, socks, or stockings can harbor microorganisms and cause offensive odors.

Cleaning and trimming nails is easier after they have been soaked. Clean under them with an orange stick. Scissors are not used to cut fingernails. Clip nails straight across with a nail clippers. Shape the nails with an emery board (Fig. 11-11). Extreme caution must be taken when clipping and trimming fingernails to prevent damage to surrounding tissues.

Nurse aides do not cut or trim toenails. Calluses and rough areas on feet should be scrubbed with a washcloth after the feet have been soaked. Lotion or petroleum jelly may be applied to feet. Broken skin or red, irritated areas should be reported to the nurse.

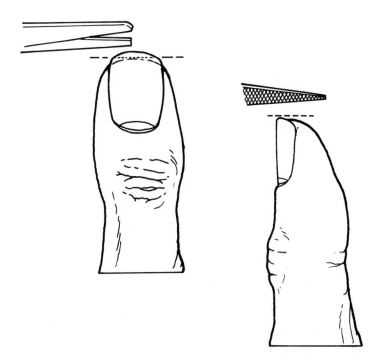

Fig. 11-11 Fingernails are clipped straight across. A nail clipper is used for this procedure. (*From Sorrentino SA:* Mosby's textbook for nursing assistants, *ed 3, St Louis, 1992, Mosby–Year Book.*)

DRESSING AND UNDRESSING RESIDENTS

Clothing changes are usually necessary on admission and discharge. Some people enter and leave the facility in a gown or pajamas. However, most wear street clothes.

Dressing and undressing occur at least daily and sometimes more often. Residents of nursing facilities wear street clothes during the day. Some residents cannot dress and undress themselves. Others need some assistance. Certain rules are followed when dressing or undressing individuals.

1. Provide for privacy. Do not expose the resident.
2. Encourage the resident to do as much as possible.
3. Remove clothing from the strong or "good" side first.
4. Put clothing on the weak side first.

CHANGING GOWNS

A resident that spends most of the time in bed will probably wear a gown. The gown is changed after a bath and when wet or soiled. Special measures are needed when there is an arm injury, paralysis, or an IV infusion. If there is an injury or paralysis, the gown is removed from the unaffected arm first. The affected arm is supported while the gown is removed. The clean gown is put on the affected arm first and then on the unaffected arm.

Some facilities have special gowns for residents receiving IV infusions. They open along the entire sleeve and are closed with ties or snaps. Traditional hospital gowns may be used for residents with IV infusions. To change the gown of a resident receiving an IV infusion, the nurse aide should untie or unsnap the gown. Remove the gown from the arm with no IV infusion. Gather up the sleeve with the IV infusion and slide it over the IV site and tubing. Remove the arm and hand from the sleeve. Gather the arm of the new gown and slide it over the arm and tubing. Remove the IV bag from the pole and slide it through the sleeve keeping it above the arm. Rehang the IV bag. Fasten the gown.

SUMMARY

Promoting cleanliness and providing hygiene are important responsibilities of the nurse aide. The resident's physical and psychological well-being are affected by good personal hygiene. Cultural and personal preferences influence the individual's hygiene practices. You should allow resident choices about hygiene.

Oral hygiene, bathing, back massages, perineal care, hair and nail care, and foot care are physically and psychologically important to the resident. Giving personal care provides a good way to get to know the resident and to observe the resident's skin condition.

CHAPTER 12

Toileting

Objectives

Identify the characteristics of normal urine
Identify the usual times for urination
Describe the general rules for maintaining normal urinary elimination
List the observations to be made about urine
Describe urinary incontinence and the care required
Explain why catheters are used
Describe the rules for caring for residents with catheters
Describe the rules for collecting urine specimens
Describe a normal stool and the normal pattern and frequency of bowel movements
List the observations about defecation that are reported to the nurse
Identify the factors that affect bowel elimination
Describe common problems relating to defecation
Describe the measures that promote comfort and safety during defecation
Explain why enemas are given
Know the common enema solutions
Describe the rules for administering enemas
Describe the purpose of a rectal tube
Describe how to care for a resident with a colostomy or ileostomy

NORMAL URINATION

The urinary system removes much of the body's waste and regulates the amount of water in the body. The kidneys, ureters, urinary bladder, and urethra are the major urinary tract structures (Fig. 12-1). Blood passes through the two kidneys, where

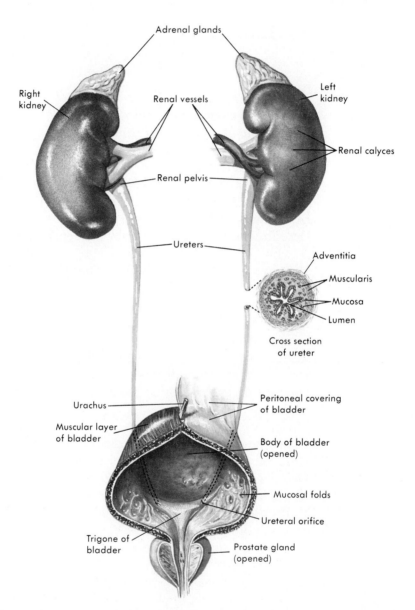

Fig. 12-1 Urinary tract structures. (*From Anderson KN, Anderson L, Glanze WD:* Mosby's medical, nursing, and allied health dictionary, *ed 3, St Louis, 1990, Mosby–Year Book.*)

urine is formed. Urine consists of the wastes and excess fluids that are filtered out of the blood. Urine flows through two ureters to the urinary bladder, where it is stored until there is a desire to urinate. The urethra is the tube that connects the urinary bladder to the outside of the body. Urine is eliminated from the body through the urethra. *Urination, micturation,* and *voiding* all mean the process of emptying the bladder.

The healthy adult excretes about 1000 to 1500 milliliters (2 to 3 pints) of urine a day. Many factors affect the amount of urine produced. These include the amount and kinds of fluid ingested, age, the amount of salt in the diet, illnesses, and drugs. Certain substances increase urine production. Examples are coffee, tea, alcohol, and some drugs. A diet high in salt causes the body to retain water. When water is retained, less urine is produced. Urine production is also influenced by body temperature, the amount of perspiration, and the external temperature.

Urinary frequency also depends on many factors. The amount of fluid ingested, personal habits, and available toilet facilities affect frequency. So do activity, work, and illness. People usually urinate at bedtime and after getting up. Some people urinate every 2 to 3 hours. Others void every 8 to 12 hours. Sleep may be disturbed if large amounts of urine are being produced.

MAINTAINING NORMAL URINATION

Residents may need help in maintaining normal elimination. Some need help getting to the bathroom. Others use bedpans, urinals, or commodes.

General rules

You need to follow these rules to help individuals maintain normal urinary elimination. The rules of medical asepsis and universal precautions are also practiced.

1. Provide a bedpan, urinal, or commode or help the person to the bathroom as soon as a request is made. The need to void may be urgent.
2. Help the person assume a normal position for voiding if possible. Women use the sitting or squatting position. Men usually stand to urinate.
3. Make sure the bedpan or urinal is warm.
4. Cover the person for warmth and privacy.
5. Provide for privacy. Pull the curtain around the bed, close doors to the room and bathroom, and pull drapes or window shades. Leave the room if the person is strong enough to be alone.
6. Remain nearby if the person is weak or unsteady.
7. Place the signal light and toilet paper within reach.
8. Allow the individual enough time to void.
9. Run water in a nearby sink or place the person's fingers in some water if the person has difficulty starting the stream.

10. Provide perineal care as needed.
11. Provide a wash basin, soap, washcloth, and towel after urination. Assist as necessary.
12. Offer the bedpan or urinal at regular intervals. Some people are embarrassed or too weak to ask.

What to report to the nurse

Before disposing of the urine, it is carefully observed. Urine is observed for color, clarity, odor, amount, and the presence of particles. Urine that looks abnormal is saved for the nurse to observe. Complaints of urgency, burning on urination, or dysuria are also reported. *Dysuria* means painful or difficult *(dys)* urination *(uria)*.

Bedpans

Bedpans are used by persons who cannot be out of bed. Women use bedpans for urination and bowel movements. Men use them for bowel movements only. Bedpans are made of plastic or stainless steel. Stainless steel bedpans tend to be cold and are warmed before being given to residents. Universal precautions should be followed and the resident's privacy maintained.

Fracture pans are also available (Fig. 12-2). A *fracture pan* has a thinner rim and is only about one-half inch deep at one end. The smaller end is placed under the buttocks. Fracture pans are used for residents with casts or those in traction.

The bedpan is covered after being used and is taken to the toilet or "dirty" utility room. After being emptied and rinsed, it is cleaned with a disinfectant. The bedpan is returned to the bedside stand with a clean cover.

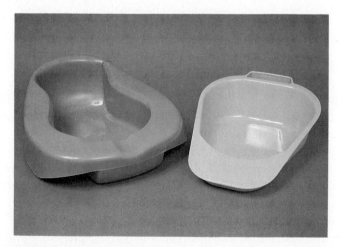

Fig. 12-2 The regular bedpan and the fracture pan. *(From Sorrentino SA:* Mosby's textbook for nursing assistants, *ed 3, St Louis, 1992, Mosby–Year Book.)*

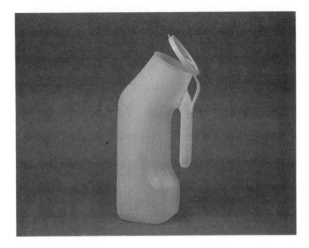

Fig. 12-3 A urinal. *(From Sorrentino SA:* Mosby's textbook for nursing assistants, *ed 3, St Louis, 1992, Mosby–Year Book.)*

Urinals

Urinals (Fig. 12-3) are used by men. They are made of the same materials as bedpans. Plastic urinals have caps at the top and hook-type handles. The hook allows the urinal to hang from the side rail within the man's reach. The urinal is used while lying in bed, sitting on the edge of the bed, or standing at the bedside. If possible, the man should stand. Some men need to be supported in the standing position. You may have to place and hold the urinal for some residents. Universal precautions should be practiced and privacy provided.

Urinals are emptied promptly to prevent odors and the spread of microorganisms. A filled urinal can easily spill and cause safety hazards. Urinals are cleaned like bedpans.

After using urinals, many men hang them on side rails or place them on nearby tables until someone empties them. This practice is to be discouraged They should be reminded to signal when urinals need to be emptied.

Commodes

A bedside commode is a portable chair or wheelchair with an opening for a bedpan or similar receptacle. Residents unable to walk to the bathroom may be allowed to use the commode. The commode lets the resident assume a normal position for elimination. The bedpan or receptacle is cleaned after use like the regular bedpan. Use good body mechanics when transferring the resident to and from the commode. Provide for safety and privacy. Follow universal precautions.

CATHETERS

A *catheter* is a rubber or plastic tube used to drain or inject fluid through a body opening. A urinary catheter is inserted through the urethra into the bladder to drain urine. An *indwelling catheter* is left in the bladder so that urine drains continuously into a drainage bag. The indwelling catheter is also called a *retention* or *Foley catheter*. A balloon near the tip is inflated after the catheter is inserted. The balloon prevents the catheter from slipping out of the bladder (Fig. 12-4). Tubing connects the catheter to the collection bag. Catheter insertion *(catheterization)* is done by a nurse or doctor. A catheter may be done for urinary incontinence.

General rules

You may care for residents with indwelling catheters. The following rules will promote their comfort and safety.

1. Make sure urine flows freely through the catheter or tubing. The tubing should not have kinks.
2. Keep the drainage bag below the level of the bladder. This prevents urine from flowing backward into the bladder. Attach the drainage bag to the bed frame.

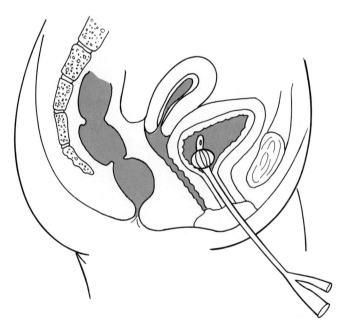

Fig. 12-4 Foley catheter. *(From Sorrentino SA:* Mosby's textbook for nursing assistants, *ed 3, St Louis, 1992, Mosby–Year Book.)*

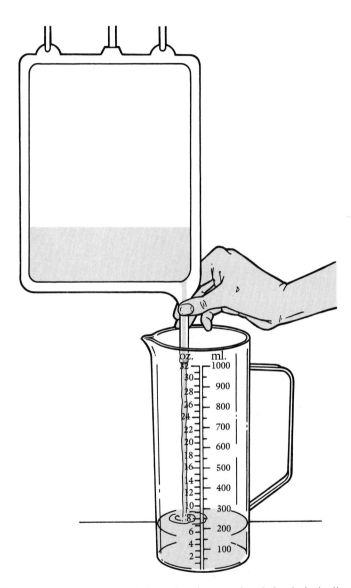

Fig. 12-5 The clamp on the urinary drainage bag is opened and the drain is directed into the graduate. *(From Sorrentino SA:* Mosby's textbook for nursing assistants, *ed 3, St Louis, 1992, Mosby–Year Book.)*

3. Coil the drainage tubing on the bed and pin it to the bottom linen. This lets urine flow freely.

4. Tape the catheter to the inner thigh or tape the catheter to the man's abdomen. This prevents excessive movement of the catheter and reduces friction at the insertion site.

5. Provide catheter care in addition to perineal care. Catheter care is done daily (8d) and may be done twice a day (bid) in some facilities. Some facilities have catheter care kits that nurse aides use. The kit contains antiseptic solution, applicators, and glove(s). To perform catheter care, provide for privacy and cover the resident. Expose the genitalia. Perform perineal care. Apply antiseptic solution to the labia or the head of the penis. Clean the catheter from the meatus (urinary opening) down for 4 inches. Use one applicator per stroke.

6. Empty the drainage bag at the end of the shift or at time intervals directed by the nurse. Measure and record the amount of urine in the bag (Fig. 12-5).

7. Report resident complaints to the nurse immediately. These include complaints of pain, burning, the need to urinate, or irritation. Also report the color, clarity, and odor of urine.

8. Follow the rules of medical asepsis and universal precautions at all times.

The condom catheter

Condom catheters (external catheter or Texas catheter) are often used for incontinent men. A condom catheter is a soft, rubber sheath that slides over the penis. Tubing connects the condom catheter and the drainage bag. Residents and home-care residents may prefer leg bags during the day.

A new condom catheter is applied daily. The penis is thoroughly washed with soap and water and dried before a new catheter is applied. Universal precautions are followed when removing or applying condom catheters.

URINARY INCONTINENCE

Urinary incontinence is the inability to control the passage of urine from the bladder. Some people dribble only when laughing, sneezing, coughing, lifting, or straining. Others dribble constantly. Some people have no control over urination. The many causes of incontinence include spinal cord injuries, central nervous system disorders, aging, and confusion. Certain medications, weak pelvic muscles, reproductive system surgery, childbirth, and urinary tract infections are also causes. Sometimes it occurs because the person cannot use the toilet, bedpan, urinal, or commode in time. A delay may be caused by difficulty in removing clothes. Incontinence may be temporary or permanent.

Incontinence is embarrassing to the person. Clothing becomes wet, odors develop, and the person is uncomfortable. Irritation, infection, and bed sores can also occur. Good skin care is essential.

COLLECTING AND TESTING URINE SPECIMENS

Urine specimens (samples) are collected for laboratory study. Urine is examined to help the doctor diagnose a problem or evaluate the effectiveness of treatment. Examples of types of urine specimens include routine, clean-catch, 24-hour, and double-voided. A laboratory requisition slip is completed for each specimen to be sent to the laboratory. The nurse is responsible for accurately completing the requisition. It has the resident's identifying information and the laboratory test to be done. Nurse aides are often asked to collect specimens.

General rules

The following rules are practiced when collecting urine specimens.

1. Wash your hands before and after collecting the specimen.
2. Use universal precautions.
3. Use a clean container for each specimen.
4. Use a container appropriate for the specimen.
5. Label the container accurately with the requested information. Most request the resident's full name, room and bed number, date, and time the specimen was collected.
6. Do not touch the inside of the container or lid.
7. Collect the specimen at the time specified.
8. The specimen must be free of fecal material.
9. Ask the resident to put toilet tissue in the toilet or wastebasket. The specimen should not contain tissue.
10. Take the specimen and requisition slip to the laboratory or designated storage place.

Routine urine specimen

The routine urine specimen is also called the random urine sample or routine urinalysis. Urine is examined for all resident's admitted to hospitals. The test is also done before surgery and for physical examinations. Many residents can collect the specimen themselves. Weak and very ill residents need assistance.

Clean-catch urine specimen

The clean-catch urine specimen is also called a midstream specimen or clean-voided specimen. The perineal area is cleaned before collecting the specimen. Perineal care reduces the number of microbes in the urethral area at the time the specimen is collected. The resident begins to void into the toilet, bedpan, urinal, or commode. Then the stream is stopped and the sterile specimen container positioned. The resident then voids into the container until the specimen is obtained.

Many people find it hard to stop the stream of urine. You may need to position and hold the specimen container in place after the resident has started to void. Be sure to wear gloves when collecting a clean-catch urine specimen and follow the principles of medical asepsis. Some facilities use clean-catch specimen kits. They are available from the supply area.

24-hour urine specimen

All urine voided during a 24-hour period is collected for a 24-hour urine specimen. Urine is chilled on ice or refrigerated during the collection period to prevent the growth of microorganisms. A preservative is added to the collection container for some tests.

The resident voids to begin the test; this voiding is discarded. *All* voidings during the next 24 hours are collected. The procedure and test period must be clearly understood by the resident and everyone involved in the resident's care. The rules for collecting urine specimens are also followed. Universal precautions are followed.

Double-voided or fresh-fractional urine specimen

A double-voided specimen is another term for a fresh-fractional urine specimen. This is because the resident voids twice. The resident voids to empty the bladder which contains "stale" urine. In 30 minutes the resident voids again. "Fresh" urine has collected in the bladder since the first voiding. The second voiding is usually a very small or "fractional" amount of urine.

Fresh-fractional specimens are used to test urine for sugar.

Testing urine

You may be responsible for testing the urine of residents with diabetes mellitus. *Diabetes mellitus* is a chronic disease in which the pancreas fails to secrete enough insulin. The insufficient amount of insulin prevents the body from using sugar for energy. Sugar builds up in the blood if it cannot be used. Some of the sugar appears in the urine. *Glucosuria* is the medical term for sugar *(glucos)* in the urine *(uria)*.

The diabetic resident may also have *acetone (ketone bodies or ketones)* in the urine. These appear in urine because of the rapid breakdown of fat for energy. Fat is used for energy because the body cannot use sugar due to the lack of insulin.

The doctor orders the type and frequency of urine tests. They are usually done four times a day: 30 minutes before each meal (ac) and at bedtime (HS or hs). The doctor uses the test results to regulate the amount of medication given. They are also used to regulate the resident's diet. You must be accurate when testing urine and promptly report the results to the nurse. Fresh-fractional urine specimens are best for testing urine for sugar and ketones.

Testape. Testape is used to test urine for sugar. A strip of tape is removed from the Testape dispenser and dipped into the specimen. Then the strip is compared to the color chart on the dispenser.

Clinitest. The Clinitest tests urine for sugar. A Clinitest tablet is added to a test tube with urine and water. The solution turns various colors depending on the amount of sugar in the urine. The Clinitest kit contains the instructions and color chart for the test. The kit is labeled with the person's name and room number. When handling urine, follow principles of medical asepsis. Place 5 drops of urine, 10 drops of water, and a Clinitest tablet in the test tube. Wait 15 seconds and compare the results to the color chart. Dispose of the contents carefully and clean the equipment. Report and record the results.

Acetest. The Acetest determines if acetone or ketone bodies are in the urine. An Acetest tablet is added to urine. The urine changes color depending on how much acetone is in the urine. Using universal precautions, place an Acetest tablet on a paper towel. Place 1 drop of urine on the tablet, wait 30 seconds, and compare to color chart. Discard the urine, tablet, and paper towel. Report and record the results.

Keto-Diastix

The Keto-Diastix (Fig. 12-6) determines if sugar and ketones (acetone) are in the urine. The plastic strip has two test areas at the bottom. The strip is dipped into a urine specimen for 2 seconds. Wait 15 seconds and then the strip is compared to a color chart. The test areas change color if sugar or ketones are present.

Straining urine. Stones (calculi) can develop in the urinary system. They may be in the kidneys, ureters, or bladder. Stones may be as small as a pin head or as large

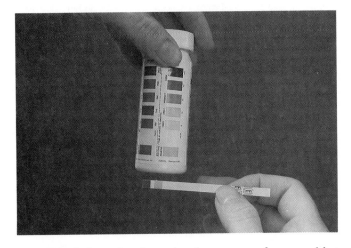

Fig. 12-6 The Keto-Diastix is used to determine the presence of sugar and ketones (acetone) in the urine. *(From Sorrentino SA:* Mosby's textbook for nursing assistants, *ed 3, St Louis, 1992, Mosby–Year Book.)*

as an orange. Stones that cause severe pain and damage to the urinary system may be removed by surgical procedures. A stone may exit the body through urine. All of the resident's urine must be strained. If a stone is passed, it is sent to the laboratory to be examined. All observations are reported to the nurse. Universal precautions are followed.

NORMAL BOWEL ELIMINATION

Bowel elimination is the excretion of wastes from the digestive system. Foods and fluids are normally taken in through the mouth and are partially digested in the stomach. The mixture of partially digested foods and fluids is called *chyme*. Chyme passes from the stomach into the small intestine. Further digestion and absorption of nutrients occurs as chyme passes through the small bowel. Chyme eventually enters the large intestine (large bowel or colon) where fluid is absorbed. There the chyme's consistency becomes less fluid and more solid. *Feces* refers to the semisolid mass of waste products in the colon.

Feces move through the intestines by *peristalsis*, the alternating contraction and

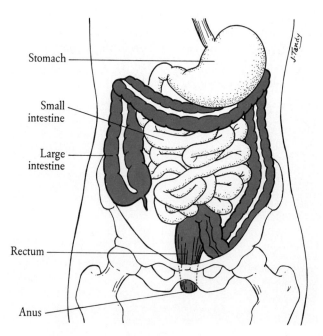

Fig. 12-7 The gastrointestinal system. (*From Sorrentino SA:* Mosby's textbook for nursing assistants, *ed 3, St Louis, 1992, Mosby–Year Book.*)

relaxation of intestinal muscles. Feces moves through the large intestine to the rectum. Feces are stored in the rectum until excreted from the body (Fig. 12-7). *Defecation (bowel movement)* is the process of excreting feces from the rectum through the anus. The term *stool* refers to feces that have been excreted.

The frequency of bowel movements is highly dependent on each person. Some people have a bowel movement every day. Others have a bowel movement every 2 to 3 days. Some people have two or three bowel movements a day. The pattern of elimination also involves the time of day. Many people defecate after breakfast, others do so in the evening.

Stools are normally brown in color. Bleeding in the stomach, intestines, or colon affects the color of stools. Color is also affected by certain disease and foods. A diet high in beets causes red-colored feces. A diet high in green vegetables can cause green stools.

Feces are normally soft, formed, and shaped like the rectum. Feces that move rapidly through the intestine are watery and unformed. This is called *diarrhea*. Stools that move slowly through the intestines are harder than normal. *Constipation* is the excretion of a hard, dry stool.

Feces have a characteristic odor. The odor is due to bacterial action in the intestines. Certain foods and drugs can affect the odor of stools.

What to report to the nurse

Stools are carefully observed before disposal. Note the color, amount, consistency, and odor. The shape and size of feces and frequency of defecation are reported. Also report any complaints of pain. Abnormal stools should be observed by the nurse.

FACTORS AFFECTING BOWEL ELIMINATION

Normal defecation is affected by many factors. Regularity, frequency, consistency, color, and odor of stools can be affected by psychological and physical factors.

Privacy

Like urination, bowel elimination is a private act. Lack of privacy may prevent a person from defecating even though the urge is felt. The odors and sounds from a bowel movement can be embarrassing. Individuals may ignore the urge to defecate to avoid having a bowel movement in the presence of others.

Diet

A well-balanced diet is important for normal bowel elimination. A certain amount of bulk is needed. Foods high in fiber are not completely digested and leave a residue that provides needed bulk. A diet low in fiber reduces the frequency of defecation, resulting in constipation. Fruits and vegetables are high in fiber.

Individual reaction to certain foods can cause diarrhea or constipation. Milk may cause constipation in some people and diarrhea in others. Chocolate and other foods can cause similar reactions.

Gas-forming foods can stimulate peristalsis. Increased peristalsis results in defecation. Gas-forming foods include onions, beans, cabbage, cauliflower, radishes, and cucumbers.

Fluids

Fecal material contains a certain amount of water. Water is absorbed from feces as it moves through the large intestine. Stool consistency depends on how much water is absorbed. The amount of fluid ingested and the amount of urine both affect the amount of water absorbed by the large intestine.

Activity

Exercise and activity maintain muscle tone and stimulate peristalsis. Irregular elimination and constipation are often due to inactivity and bed rest. Inactivity may result from disease, surgery, injury, and aging.

Medications

Medications can prevent constipation or control diarrhea. Other medications, unrelated to bowel elimination, may have the side effects of diarrhea or constipation. Drugs for pain relief often cause constipation. Antibiotics, used to fight or prevent infection, often cause diarrhea. Diarrhea results because antibiotics kill the normal bacteria in the large intestine. Normal bacteria are necessary for the formation of stool.

COMMON PROBLEMS

Many factors can affect normal bowel elimination. Common problems include constipation, fecal impaction, diarrhea, anal incontinence, and flatulence.

Constipation

Constipation is the passage of a hard, dry stool. The person usually strains to have a bowel movement. The stool may be large or marble-sized. Large stools cause pain as they pass through the anus. Constipation occurs when feces move through the intestine slowly, allowing more time for the absorption of water. Common causes of constipation include ignoring the urge to defecate, diet, decreased fluid intake, inactivity, medications, aging, and certain diseases.

Fecal impaction

A *fecal impaction* is the prolonged retention and accumulation of feces in the rectum. Fecal material is hard or puttylike in consistency. A fecal impaction results if constipation is not relieved. The person cannot defecate and more water is absorbed from the already hardened feces. Liquid seeping from the anus is a sign of fecal impaction. Liquid feces pass around the hardened fecal mass in the rectum.

The person with a fecal impaction may try several times to have a bowel movement. Abdominal discomfort and rectal pain may be reported. The doctor may order medications and enemas to remove the impaction. The nurse may have to remove the fecal mass with a lubricated, gloved finger.

Diarrhea

Diarrhea is the frequent passage of liquid stools. Feces move through the intestines rapidly, reducing the time for fluid absorption. There is an urgent need to defecate. Some people have difficulty maintaining control of elimination. Abdominal cramping, nausea, and vomiting may also occur.

Causes of diarrhea include infections, certain medications, irritating foods, and microorganisms in food and water. Medical treatment involves reducing peristalsis by diet or medications. You must provide the bedpan or commode promptly for a person with diarrhea. Prompt disposal of the stool is necessary to reduce odors and prevent the spread of microorganisms. Good skin care is essential. Liquid feces is very irritating to the skin. So is the frequent wiping of the anal area with toilet tissue. Sores may develop if cleanliness and good skin care are not practiced. Principles of good medical asepsis must be followed.

Anal incontinence

Anal incontinence (fecal incontinence) is the inability to control the passage of feces and gas through the anus. Diseases or injuries to the nervous system may cause anal incontinence. Sometimes it results from an unanswered signal light when the person needs the bedpan or help getting to the commode or bathroom.

The person with anal incontinence needs good skin care. A bowel training program may be developed. Providing the bedpan or commode after meals or every 2 to 3 hours may be helpful. Consider the psychological impact of anal incontinence on the person. Frustration, embarrassment, anger, and humiliation are a few of the emotions experienced.

Flatulence

Gas or air in the stomach or intestines is called *flatus*. Swallowing air while eating and drinking and bacterial action in the intestines are common sources of flatus. Normally flatus is expelled through the mouth and anus.

Flatulence is the excessive formation of gas in the stomach and intestines. If the gas is not expelled the intestines distend. In other words, they swell or enlarge from the pressure of the gases. The person may have abdominal cramping, shortness of breath, and a swollen abdomen. Flatulence may be caused by gas-forming foods, constipation, medications, and abdominal surgery. In addition, tense or anxious people may swallow large amounts of air when drinking. Doctors may prescribe enemas, medications, or rectal tubes to relieve distention.

COMFORT AND SAFETY DURING ELIMINATION

Certain measures help promote normal bowel elimination. The nurse plans measures that involve diet, fluids, and exercise. The following actions should be routinely practiced to promote bowel elimination, comfort, and safety.

1. Provide the bedpan or help the patient to the toilet or commode as soon as it is requested.
2. Provide for privacy. Ask visitors to leave the room. Close doors, pull curtains around the bed, and pull window curtains or shades.
3. Make sure the bedpan is warm.
4. Position the person in a normal sitting position.
5. Make sure the person is adequately covered for warmth and privacy.
6. Allow enough time for defecation.
7. Place the signal light and toilet tissue within the person's reach.
8. Stay nearby if the person is weak or unsteady.
9. Provide perineal care.
10. Dispose of feces promptly. This reduces odors and prevents the spread of microorganisms.
11. Let the person wash their hands after defecating and wiping with toilet tissue.
12. Offer the bedpan after meals if the person has the problem of incontinence.
13. Use universal precautions if contact with feces is possible.

ENEMAS

An *enema* is the introduction of fluid into the rectum and lower colon. Enemas are ordered by doctors. They are given to remove feces and to relieve constipation or fecal impaction. They are also ordered to clean the bowel of feces before certain surgeries, x-ray procedures, or childbirth. Sometimes enemas are ordered to remove flatus and relieve intestinal distention.

Enema solutions

The enema solution ordered by the doctor depends on the purpose of the enema. The solution may be *tap water* obtained from a faucet. A *soap solution* enema (SSE) is prepared by adding 5 milliliters (ml) of liquid soap to 1000 ml of water. A *saline* enema is a solution of salt and water. These solutions are generally used for cleansing enemas. Cleansing enemas involve the removal of feces from the rectum and colon.

Oil is used for oil retention enemas. They are given for constipation or fecal impactions. The oil is retained in the rectum for 30 to 60 minutes to soften the feces and lubricate the rectum. This allows feces to pass with ease. Mineral oil, olive oil, or a commercial oil retention enema may be used.

Commercial enemas are often ordered for constipated residents. They are also ordered when complete cleansing of the bowel is not indicated. The enema contains about 120 ml (4 ounces) of a solution. It causes defecation by irritating and distending the rectum.

Other enema solutions may be ordered. Consult with the nurse and use the procedure manual to safely prepare and give uncommon enemas.

Equipment

Disposable enema kits are available. The kit (Fig. 12-8) includes a plastic enema bag, tubing, a clamp for the tubing, and a waterproof bed protector. The enema bag holds the solution. Most kits have packets of castile soap for soap sud enemas. Lu-

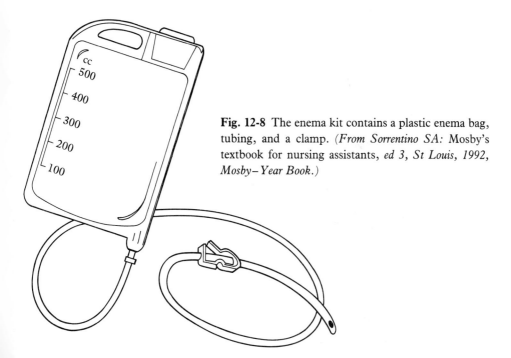

Fig. 12-8 The enema kit contains a plastic enema bag, tubing, and a clamp. *(From Sorrentino SA:* Mosby's textbook for nursing assistants, *ed 3, St Louis, 1992, Mosby–Year Book.)*

bricant is needed if the tubing end is not prelubricated. A bath thermometer is used to measure the temperature of the solution. If a commercial enema has been ordered, you need the enema kit and a waterproof bed protector. A bedpan or commode is usually needed for an enema. Enema procedures also require gloves for universal precautions.

General rules

The administration of an enema is generally a safe procedure. Many people give themselves enemas at home. However, enemas are dangerous for people with certain heart and kidney diseases. Give an enema only after receiving clear instructions and after reviewing the procedure with the nurse.

Comfort and safety measures are practiced when giving an enema. In addition, these rules must be followed.

1. Solution temperature should be 105° F (40.5° C). Measure the temperature with a bath thermometer.
2. The amount of solution to be given depends on the enema's purpose and the person's age. Adults generally receive 750 to 1000 ml.
3. The left Sim's position is usually used (Fig. 12-9). However, a comfortable left side-lying position may be allowed.
4. The enema bag is raised no more than 18 inches above the level of the mattress.
5. The lubricated enema tubing is inserted only 2 to 4 inches into the rectum. The intestine can be injured if the tube is inserted any deeper.
6. The solution is administered slowly. Usually it takes 10 to 15 minutes to give 750 to 1000 ml.
7. The solution should be retained in the bowel for a certain length of time. The length of time depends on the amount and type of solution.
8. The enema tube is held in place while the solution is being administered.
9. Have the bedpan or commode ready or, if the bathroom is going to be used, make sure the bathroom is vacant when the person has the urge to defecate.
10. The nurse is asked to observe the results of the enema.
11. Universal precautions are used.

The cleansing enema

Cleansing enemas are often given to clean the bowel of feces and flatus. They are sometimes given before surgery, x-ray procedures, and childbirth. The doctor may order a soap solution, tap water, or saline enema. The doctor may order "enemas until clear." Enemas are given until the return solution is clear and free of fecal material. Check with the nurse to see how many enemas can be given. The facility may only allow enemas to be repeated two or three times.

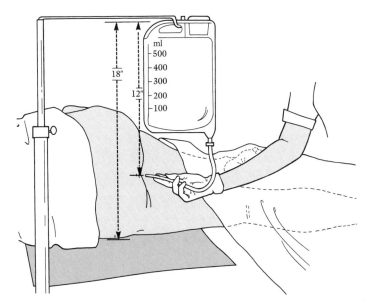

Fig. 12-9 The left Sim's position. (*From Sorrentino SA:* Mosby's textbook for nursing assistants, *ed 3, St Louis, 1992, Mosby–Year Book.)*

Tap water enemas can be dangerous. The large intestine may absorb some of the water into the bloodstream. This creates a fluid imbalance in the body. Repeated enemas increase the risk of excessive fluid absorption. Soap solution enemas are very irritating to the bowel's mucous lining. Damage to the bowel can result with repeated enemas. Using more than 5 ml of castile soap and using stronger soaps can also damage the bowel. The saline enema solution is similar to body fluid. However, some people may absorb some of the salt that is in the solution.

To give an enema, place the resident in left Sim's position. Insert the enema tube into the rectum and give the fluid slowly. Instruct the resident to take deep breaths. Give the desired amount of fluid or the amount the resident can tolerate. Assist the resident to the commode or onto the bedpan. Provide for safety. Report and record results and clean the equipment.

The commercial enema

The commercial enema is ready to be given (Fig. 12-10). The solution is usually given at room temperature. However, the nurse may have you warm the enema in a basin of warm water. The left Sim's or a left side-lying position is often used.

The plastic bottle is squeezed and rolled up from the bottom to administer the solution (Fig. 12-11). Squeezing and rolling are continued until all solution has been

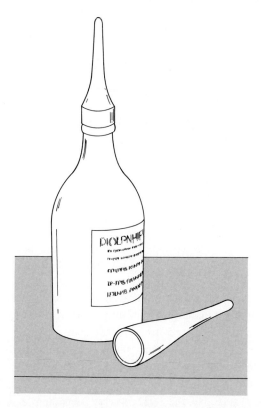

Fig. 12-10 A commercially prepared enema. (*From Sorrentino SA:* Mosby's textbook for nursing assistants, *ed 3, St Louis, 1992, Mosby–Year Book.*)

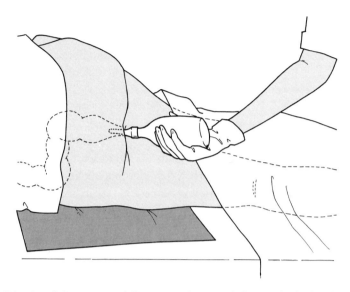

Fig. 12-11 The tip of the commercially prepared enema is inserted 2 inches into the rectum. (*From Sorrentino SA:* Mosby's textbook for nursing assistants, *ed 3, St Louis, 1992, Mosby–Year Book.*)

given. Do not release pressure on the bottle. If pressure is released, solution is withdrawn from the rectum back into the bottle. Encourage the resident to retain the solution until the urge to defecate is felt. Remaining in the Sim's or side-lying position will help the person retain the enema longer. Assist the resident to the commode or place the resident on the bedpan. Provide for the resident's comfort and safety.

The oil retention enema

Commercial oil retention enemas are administered like other commercial enemas. However, the solution is retained in the rectum so the feces soften. The enema is retained for a specified length of time, usually for 30 to 60 minutes. Oil retention enemas are ordered to relieve constipation or fecal impaction.

THE RESIDENT WITH AN OSTOMY

Cancer, diseases of the bowel, and trauma are common reasons for intestinal surgery. An ostomy may be necessary. An *ostomy* is the surgical creation of an artificial opening. The opening is called the *stoma*. The nurse may need your assistance in giving postoperative care, or you may care for a person who has had an ostomy for a long time.

Colostomy

A *colostomy* is the surgical creation of an artificial opening between the colon and abdomen. Part of the colon is brought out onto the abdominal wall and a stoma is made. Feces and flatus pass through the stoma rather than the anus. Colostomies may be permanent or temporary. If permanent, the diseased part of the colon is removed. A temporary colostomy gives the diseased or injured bowel time to heal. After healing occurs, surgery is done to reconnect the bowel.

The colostomy location depends on the part of the colon that is diseased or injured (Fig. 12-12). Stool consistency depends on the location of the colostomy. The more colon that is remaining to absorb water, the more solid and formed the stool. If the colostomy is near the beginning of the colon, stools will be liquid in consistency. A colostomy near the end of the large intestine results in formed stools.

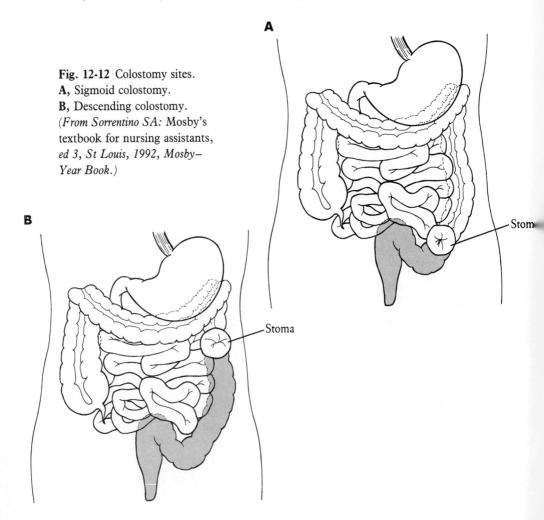

Fig. 12-12 Colostomy sites.
A, Sigmoid colostomy.
B, Descending colostomy.
(*From Sorrentino SA:* Mosby's textbook for nursing assistants, *ed 3, St Louis, 1992, Mosby– Year Book.*)

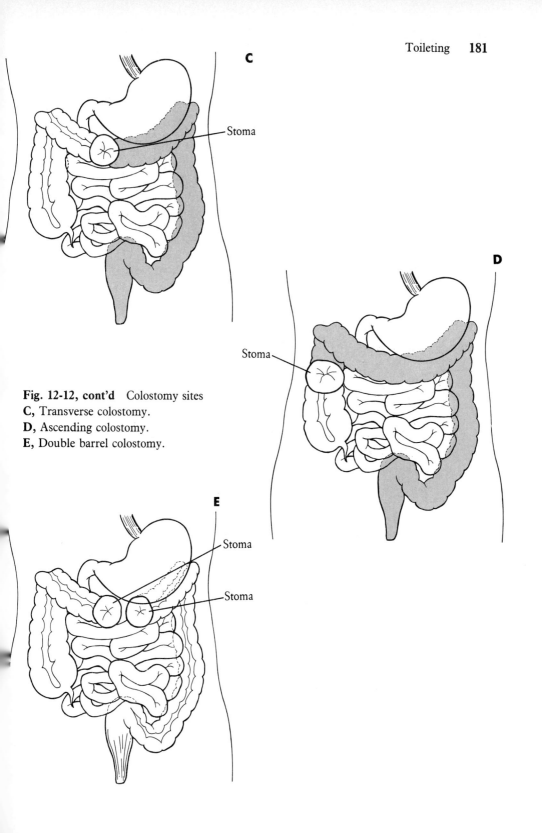

Fig. 12-12, cont'd   Colostomy sites
C, Transverse colostomy.
D, Ascending colostomy.
E, Double barrel colostomy.

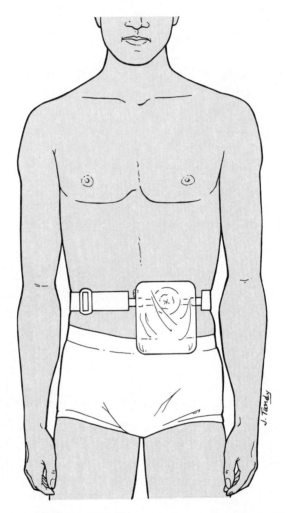

Fig. 12-13 A colostomy appliance is in place over the stoma and secured with a colostomy belt. *(From Sorrentino SA:* Mosby's textbook for nursing assistants, *ed 3, St Louis, 1992, Mosby–Year Book.)*

The individual wears a colostomy appliance (Fig. 12-13). The appliance is a disposable plastic bag applied over the stoma. It collects feces expelled through the stoma. When the appliance becomes soiled, it is removed and a new one applied. Skin care is given to prevent skin breakdown around the stoma. The appliance has an adhesive backing that is applied to the skin. Many people also secure the appliance to an ostomy belt. Many people manage their colostomies without assistance. If able, they are allowed to do so in the health-care facility.

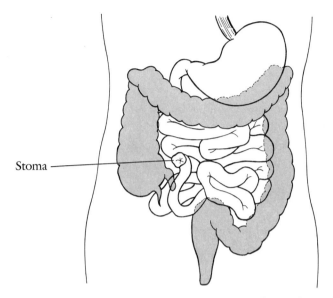

Stoma

Fig. 12-14 An ileostomy. *(From Sorrentino SA:* Mosby's textbook for nursing assistants, *ed 3, St Louis, 1992, Mosby–Year Book.)*

Odors need to be prevented. Good hygiene is essential. A new bag is applied whenever soiling occurs. Emptying the bag of feces and avoiding gas-forming foods also help to control odors. Special deodorants can be put into the appliance. The nurse will tell you which one to use.

To replace a colostomy bag, the nurse aide uses universal precautions and gently removes the colostomy belt and bag. Place it in a bedpan or bag. Gently wipe with tissue around the stoma. Cleanse and rinse the area around the stoma and pat dry. Apply a skin barrier (karaya powder, karaya ring, or other barrier). Apply a new appliance after removing the adhesive. Reapply the belt. Discard the appliance after observing and reporting characteristics of the stool to the nurse. Use the principles of medical asepsis.

Ileostomy

An *ileostomy* is the surgical creation of an artificial opening between the ileum (small intestine) and the abdomen. Part of the ileum is brought out onto the abdominal wall and a stoma is made. The entire large intestine is removed (Fig. 12-14). Liquid feces drain constantly from a ileostomy. Water is not absorbed because the colon has been removed. Feces in the small intestine contain digestive juices and are very irritating to the skin. The ileostomy appliance must fit well so feces do not

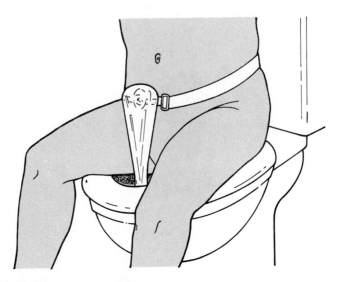

Fig. 12-15 The resident with the ileostomy empties the appliance by directing it into the toilet and unclamping the end. *(From Sorrentino SA:* Mosby's textbook for nursing assistants, *ed 3, St Louis, 1992, Mosby–Year Book.)*

touch the skin. The appliance is sealed to the skin and is removed every 2 to 4 days. Good skin care is essential.

There are disposable and reusable ileostomy appliances. The appliance is clamped at the end so feces collect in the bag. To empty the bag, direct it into the toilet and remove the clamp (Fig. 12-15). The appliance is emptied every 4 to 6 hours (q4h to q6h) or when the person urinates. Reusable bags are washed with soap and water and allowed to dry and air out. The care of a resident with an ileostomy is similar to that of a resident with a colostomy.

COLLECTING STOOL SPECIMENS

Stool specimens are sent to the laboratory. When internal bleeding is suspected, feces are checked for the presence of blood. Stools are also studied for fat, microorganisms, worms, and other abnormal contents. The rules for collecting urine specimens apply when collecting stool specimens. So do universal precautions. Assist the resident onto the bedpan or commode. After the resident has defecated, transfer the resident off the commode. The stool is obtained using a tongue blade. Place the specimen into a container and label correctly.

The stool specimen must not be contaminated with urine. Some tests require a warm stool. The specimen is taken to the laboratory immediately if a warm stool is needed. Assist the resident with perineal care as needed and provide for privacy and safety. Report and record the results to the charge nurse.

SUMMARY

You are responsible for assisting the residents to maintain normal urination. You also assist with bladder training, collecting specimens, and test urine for sugar and acetone. You must follow the rules of medical asepsis, universal precautions, cleanliness, and skin care. Your observations of the person's urine are valuable to doctors and nurses. They use your observations to plan and evaluate the person's treatment and progress.

Position and privacy are important for urinary elimination. Urination is considered a private function. Voiding is easier and more comfortable if the person can urinate in a normal position and in private.

Your responsibilities in assisting individuals with bowel elimination are similar to those for urinary elimination. The act of defecation is private. Bowel control is important to people, as are the hygiene practices that follow bowel movements. Well-being is closely associated with maintaining normal bowel function. The personal routines related to defecation also affect well-being.

Normal bowel elimination is not always possible. Constipation, fecal impaction, diarrhea, anal incontinence, and flatuence are common problems. The doctor may order enemas, rectal tubes, medications, or dietary changes to relieve the problem. The nurse may direct you to give an enema. The instructions and procedures must be thoroughly understood. Ileostomies or colostomies are sometimes necessary to treat bowel problems.

When assisting the person with bowel elimination, always consider the person's need for privacy and bowel control. The person's dignity and psychological well-being are just as important as the physical act of defecation. In addition, the rules of medical asepsis, universal precautions, cleanliness, skin care, and safety must be followed.

CHAPTER 13

Feeding Techniques

Objectives

Define nutrition.

Identify the foods found in the four basic food groups.

Explain the importance of protein, carbohydrates, and fats in the diet.

Identify major sources of proteins, carbohydrates, and fats.

Describe functions of vitamins and minerals.

Identify the dietary sources of vitamins and minerals.

Describe special diets.

Identify the nurse aide's role in caring for residents requiring special or therapeutic diets.

Describe a normal adult's daily fluid requirements.

Explain the purpose of and how to measure intake and output.

Explain the procedure for feeding a resident.

Food and water are basic physical needs that are necessary for life and health. The amount and quality of foods and fluids in the diet are important. They influence an individual's current and future physical and psychological well-being. A poor diet and poor eating habits make a person more susceptible to infection and development of chronic diseases. Healing difficulties and abnormalities in body functions are also related to poor diet and eating habits. Poor physical and mental functioning make an individual more prone to accidents and injuries. Besides being necessary for survival, eating and drinking provide pleasure. They are associated with social activities with family and friends.

Dietary practices are influenced by many factors, including culture, finances, and personal preference. These practices include selection of food and the way it is prepared and served. The role of the nursing aide in meeting a resident's needs for food and fluids is presented in this unit.

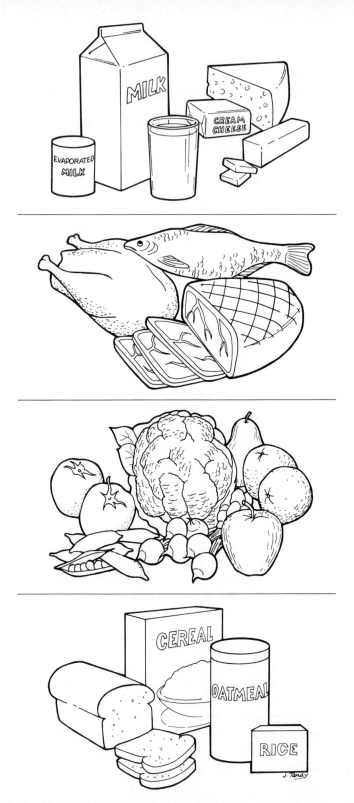

Fig. 13-1 The four basic food groups. (*From Sorrentino SA:* Mosby's textbook for nursing assistants, *ed 3, St Louis, 1992, Mosby–Year Book.*)

NUTRITION

The term "nutrition" has been defined in several ways. Essentially, nutrition is the many processes involved in the ingestion, digestion, absorption, and use of foods and fluids by the body. Good nutrition is needed for growth, healing, and maintaining body functions. It begins with the proper selection of foods and fluids. They need to be selected to provide a well-balanced diet and appropriate caloric intake. A diet that includes many foods high in calories will result in excessive weight gain or obesity. The inadequate intake of calories results in weight loss.

Foods and fluids contain nutrients. A nutrient is a substance that is ingested, digested, absorbed, and used by the body. Nutrients are grouped into the categories of fats, proteins, carbohydrates, vitamins, and minerals. The essential nutrients are found in the four basic food groups.

Fats, proteins, and carbohydrates provide the body with fuel for energy. The amount of energy provided by a nutrient is measured in calories. A calorie is the amount of energy produced from the burning of food by the body. Energy is needed for all body functions. Even sitting in a chair requires energy. The amount of calories needed by a person depends on many factors. These include age, sex, activity, climate, state of health, and the amount of sleep obtained.

Food groups

There are four basic food groups. They are milk and dairy products, meats and fish, fruits and vegetables, and breads and cereals (Fig. 13-1). The essential nutrients are found in varying amounts in each group. A well-balanced daily diet includes the recommended number of servings from each food group and all of the essential nutrients. Usually the daily diet includes three regular meals.

Milk and dairy products. The main nutrients found in milk and daily products are protein, fat, carbohydrates, calcium, and riboflavin. Milk and foods or fluids made from whole or skimmed milk (cheese and ice cream) are included in this group.

Meats and fish. Protein, fat, iron, and thiamin are the main nutrients found in meats and fish. An individual should have two or more servings daily from this group. The meat and fish group includes beef, veal, lamb, poultry, pork, fish, eggs, and cheese. Alternatives or substitutes for meat and fish are dry beans, peas, nuts, and peanut butter.

The serving size is important when planning a well-balanced diet. This is especially important for meat and fish because they contain a high number of calories. Serving size is influenced by many factors, including culture, appetite, personal preference, and the recipe used.

Fruits and vegetables. Vitamins A and C, carbohydrates, and small amounts of other nutrients are found in fruits and vegetables. Four or more servings of this food group should be part of the daily diet. This group includes fruits, dark green and yellow vegetables, tomatoes, potatoes, and fruit and vegetable juices.

Breads and cereals. Four or more servings of bread and cereal are needed daily for a well-balanced diet. Protein, carbohydrates, iron, thiamin, niacin, and riboflavin are the main nutrients found in this group. Food included in this group are bread, cereal, pasta, and crackers.

NUTRIENTS

No one food or food group contains all the essential nutrients needed by the body. A well-balanced diet consists of servings from each of the four basic food groups. It ensures an adequate intake of the essential nutrients. The major classifications of nutrients and their functions in the body are presented in this section. Also presented are the foods that contain these nutrients.

Protein

Protein is the most important nutrient—it is needed for tissue growth and repair. One gram (g) of protein provides the body with 4 calories. The sources of protein include meat, fish, poultry, eggs, milk and milk products, cereals, beans, peas, and nuts. Foods high in protein are generally the most expensive. Therefore, protein is often lacking in the diets of people with low incomes.

Every cell in the body is made up of protein. Excessive protein intake results in some protein excreted in the urine. Some will be changed into body fat and some into carbohydrates. Carbohydrates are stored in the liver.

Carbohydrates

Carbohydrates provide the body with energy. They also provide fiber for bowel elimination. Carbohydrates are found in fruits, vegetables, breads, cereals, and sugar. These foods are rather inexpensive. Rarely are carbohydrates lacking in the diet. One gram of carbohydrate provides 4 calories.

Carbohydrates are broken down into sugars during the digestive process. The sugars are then absorbed into the bloodstream. The fiber in foods containing carbohydrates is not digested. It provides the bulky part of chyme in the elimination process. Excess carbohydrate intake results in some of the nutrient being stored in the liver. The remainder is changed into body fat.

Fats

Fats also provide the body with energy. One gram of fat provides 9 calories. Besides being a source of energy, fats serve many functions in the body. They enhance the taste of food and help the body use certain vitamins. Fats also conserve body heat and protect organs from injury. The dietary sources of fat include the fat in meats, lard, butter, shortenings, salad and vegetable oils, milk, cheese, egg yolks, and nuts. These sources are more expensive than carbohydrate sources. Dietary fat not needed by the body is stored as body fat.

Vitamins

Although they do not provide calories in significant amounts, vitamins are essential nutrients. They are ingested through food and cannot be produced by the body. Vitamins A, D, E, and K can be stored by the body. Vitamin C and the B-complex vitamins are not stored and must be ingested daily. Each vitamin is necessary for specific body functions. The lack of a particular vitamin results in signs and symptoms of a particular disease. Table 5 summarizes the sources and major functions of common vitamins.

Minerals

A well-balanced diet supplies the necessary amounts of minerals. Minerals are involved in various body processes. They are needed for bone and teeth formation, nerve and muscle function, fluid balance, and other body processes. Table 6 summarizes the major functions and dietary sources of common minerals.

Factors that affect eating and nutrition

Nutrition and eating habits are influenced by many factors. Some of the factors begin during infancy and continue throughout life. Others develop later. The major influences on eating and nutrition are culture, religion, appetite, finances, personal preference, and illness.

SPECIAL DIETS

Doctors may prescribe special diets for some individuals. A special diet may be ordered because of a nutritional deficiency, a disease, or to eliminate or decrease certain substances in the diet. Special diets may be prescribed for weight control. The doctor, nurses, and dietician work together to meet the resident's nutritional needs. They will consider the need for dietary changes, personal preferences, religion, culture, and eating problems.

Many residents do not require special diets. General diet is the term used in many health-care facilities when there are no dietary restrictions or modifications. Special or therapeutic diets may be ordered for residents with diabetes, diseases of the heart, kidneys, gallbladder, liver, stomach, or intestines. Allergies, obesity, and other disorders also require therapeutic diets. Table 7 summarizes the common therapeutic diets.

The sodium-restricted diet and diabetic diet are commonly ordered. Nurse aides working in health-care facilities are likely to encounter these diets.

Table 5 Major functions and sources of common vitamins

Vitamin	Major functions	Sources
A	Growth; vision; healthy hair, skin, and mucous membranes; resistance to infection	Liver, spinach, green leafy and yellow vegetables, fruits, fish liver oils, egg yolk, butter, cream, milk
B_1 (Thiamin)	Muscle tone; nerve function; digestion; appetite; normal elimination; use of carbohydrates	Pork, liver and other organ meats, breads and cereals, potatoes, peas, beans, and soybeans
B_2 (Riboflavin)	Growth; healthy eyes, protein and carbohydrate metabolism; healthy skin and mucous membranes	Milk and milk products, organ meats, green leafy vegetables, eggs, breads and cereals
B_3 (Niacin) .	Protein, fat, and carbohydrate metabolism; functioning of the nervous system; appetite; functioning of the digestive system	Meat, poultry, fish, peanut butter, breads and cereals, peas and beans, eggs, liver
B_{12}	Formation of red blood cells; protein metabolism; functioning of the nervous system	Liver and other organ meats, meats, fish, eggs, green leafy vegetables
Folic acid	Formation of red blood cells, functioning of the intestines, protein metabolism	Liver, meats, fish, yeast, green leafy vegetables, eggs, mushrooms
C	Formation of substances that hold tissues together; healthy blood vessels, skins, gums, bones, and teeth; wound healing; prevention of bleeding; resistance to infection	Citrus fruits, tomatoes, potatoes, cabbage, strawberries, green vegetables, melons
D	Absorption and metabolism of calcium and phosphorus; healthy bones	Fish liver oils, milk, butter, liver, exposure to sunlight
E	Normal reproduction; formation of red blood cells, muscle function	Vegetable oils, milk, eggs, meats, fish, cereals, green leafy vegetables
K	Blood clotting	Liver, green leafy vegetables, margarine, soybean and vegetable oils, eggs

Sodium-restricted diet

The average amount of sodium in the daily diet is 3000 to 5000 milligrams (mg). Sodium is found in table salt and many foods. The body only needs half this amount daily. Healthy people excrete excess sodium in the urine. However, heart and kidney disease cause the body to retain the extra sodium.

Sodium-restricted diets are usually ordered for patients with heart disease. They may also be ordered for persons with liver disease, kidney disease, certain complications of pregnancy, and when certain medications are being taken. Sodium causes the body to retain water. If there is too much sodium in the body, the body retains more water. Body tissues swell with water and there are excess amounts of fluid in the blood vessels. The increased fluid in the body tissues and bloodstream forces the heart to work harder. In other words, the workload of the heart is increased. In the presence of heart disease, the extra workload can cause severe complications or death. By restricting the amount of sodium in the diet, the amount of sodium in the body is decreased. Therefore, the body retains less water. Less water in the tissues and blood vessels reduces the amount of work the heart has to perform.

There are five levels of sodium-restricted diets. The levels range from mild to severe. The doctor orders the amount of restriction appropriate for the resident.

Text continued on p. 198.

Table 6 Major functions and sources of common minerals

Mineral	Major functions	Sources
Calcium	Formation of teeth and bones; blood clotting;; muscle contraction; heart function; nerve function	Milk and milk products, green leafy vegetables
Phosphorus	Formation of bones and teeth; use of proteins, fats, and carbohydrates; nerve muscle function	Meat, fish, poultry, milk and milk products, nuts, eggs
Iron	Allows red blood cells to carry oxygen	Liver and other organ meats, egg yolks, green leafy vegetables, breads and cereals
Iodine	Thyroid gland function, growth, and metabolism	Iodized salt, seafood and shellfish, vegetables
Sodium	Fluid balance; nerve and muscle function	Almost all foods
Potassium	Nerve function; muscle contraction; heart function	Fruits, vegetables, cereals, coffee, meats

Table 7 Common therapeutic diets

Diet and description	Use	Foods allowed
Clear-liquid Clear liquids that do not leave a residue; nonirritating and not gas-forming	Post-operatively; for acute illness and nausea and vomiting	Water, tea, and coffee (without milk or cream); carbonated beverages; gelatin; clear fruit juices (apple, grape, and cranberry); fat-free clear broth; hard candy, sugar, and popsicles
Full-liquid Foods that are liquid at room temperature or that melt at body temperature	Advance from clear-liquid diet; post-operatively, for stomach irritation, fever, and nausea and vomiting	All foods allowed on a clear liquid; custard; eggnog; strained soups; strained fruit and vegetable juices; milk; creamed cereals, ice cream and sherbert
Soft Semisolid foods that are easily digested	Advance from full-liquid diet; for chewing difficulties, gastrointestinal disorders, and infections	All liquids; eggs (not fried); broiled, baked, or roasted meat, fish, or poultry; mild cheeses (American, Swiss, cheddar, cream, and cottage); strained or refined bread and crackers; cooked or pureed vegetables; cooked or canned fruit without skin or seeds; pudding; and plain cakes

Low-residue
Food that leaves a small amount of residue in the colon

For disease of the colon and diarrhea

Coffee, tea, milk, carbonated beverages, strained fruit juices; refined bread and crackers; creamed and refined cereal; rice; cottage and cream cheese; eggs (not fried); plain puddings and cakes; gelatin; custard; sherbert and ice cream; strained vegetable juices; canned or cooked fruit without skin or seeds; potatoes (not fried); strained cooked vegetables and plain pasta

High-residue
Foods that increase the amount of residue in the colon to stimulate peristalsis

For constipation and colon disorders

All fruits and vegetables; whole wheat bread; whole grain cereals; fried foods; whole grain rice; milk, cream, butter, and cheese; and meats

High-iron
Foods that are high in iron

For anemia; following blood loss; for women during the reproductive years

Liver and other organ meats; lean meats; egg yolks; shellfish; dried fruits; dried beans; green leafy vegetables; lima beans; peanut butter; and enriched breads and cereals

Continued.

Table 7 Common therapeutic diets cont'd

Diet and description	Use	Foods allowed
Bland		
Foods that are mechanically and chemically nonirritating and low in roughage; foods served at moderate temperatures; strong spices and condiments are avoided	For ulcers, gallbladder disorders, and some intestinal disorders; postoperatively following abdominal surgery	Lean meats; white bread; creamed and refined cereals; cream or cottage cheese; gelatin, plain puddings, cakes, and cookies; eggs (not fried); butter and cream; canned fruits and vegetables without skin and seeds; strained fruit juices; potatoes (not fried); pastas and rice; strained or soft cooked carrots, peas, beets, spinach, squash, and asparagus tips; creamed soups from allowed vegetables; no fried foods are allowed
High-calorie		
The numbers of calories is increased to approximately 4000; includes three full meals and between-meal snacks	For weight gain and some thyroid imbalances	Dietary increases in all foods

Low-calorie
The number of calories is reduced below the minimum daily requirements

For weight reduction

Foods low in fats and carbohydrates and lean meats; avoid butter, cream, rice, gravies, salad oils, noodles, cakes, pastries, carbonated and alcoholic beverages, candy, potato chips, and similar foods

Low-fat (low-cholesterol)
Protein and carbohydrates are increased with a limited amount of fat in the diet

For heart disease, gall-bladder disease, disorders of fat digestion, and liver disease

Skimmed milk or buttermilk; cottage cheese (no other cheeses are allowed); gelatin; sherbert; fruit; lean meat, poultry, and fish (baked, broiled, or roasted); fat-free broth; soups made with skimmed milk; margarine; rice, pasta, breads and cereals, vegetables; and potatoes

High-protein
Protein is increased to aid and promote tissue healing

For burns, high fever, infection, and some liver diseases

Meat, milk, eggs, cheese, fish, poultry; breads and cereals; and green leafy vegetables

Diabetic
The amount of carbohydrates and number of calories are regulated; protein and fat are also regulated

For diabetes mellitus

Determined by nutritional and energy requirements

Diabetic diet

The diabetic diet is ordered for residents with diabetes mellitus. Diabetes mellitus is a chronic disease in which there is a deficiency of insulin in the body. Insulin is produced and secreted by the pancreas and is needed for the body to use sugar. If there is not enough insulin, sugar builds up in the bloodstream rather than being used by body cells for energy. Diabetes is usually treated with insulin therapy, diet, and exercise.

As stated earlier, carbohydrates are broken down into sugar during the process of digestion. The amount of carbohydrates is controlled with the diabetic diet. By controlling the amount of carbohydrates, the person will take in the amount needed by the body. Excess carbohydrates are eliminated so the body does not have to use or store them. Therefore, the diabetic diet involves the amount and right kind of food for the resident.

The doctor determines how much carbohydrate, fat, protein, and calories an individual should have. Sex, activity, and weight are considered when deciding the resident's diet.

The calories and nutrients allowed are divided among three meals and between-meal nourishments. The resident must eat only what is allowed and all that is allowed. This is important so that the resident does not get too many or too few carbohydrates. The American Diabetes Association provides lists of foods that have equal value in terms of nutrients and calories provided. The foods are divided into six categories: milk, vegetables, fruits, meat, foods, and fat. The six groups are referred to as "exchanges lists" or "exchanges". The exchanges allow for variety in menu planning. For example, if a resident may not want to eat a grapefruit, he or she can look over the exchange list for fruits and find something more appealing, such as an orange. The nurse and dietitian teach the resident and family to use the exchange lists.

You need to make sure that the resident's meal is served on time. The resident with diabetes must eat at regular intervals to maintain a certain blood sugar.

It's important for the diabetic resident to eat all that is served. If not, a between-meal nourishment may be needed.

FLUID BALANCE

Except for oxygen, water is the most important physical need for survival. Death can result from an inadequate intake of water or from the excessive loss of fluid from the body. Water is obtained by taking in food and fluids.

Water is lost through the urine and feces, through the skin as perspiration, and through the lungs with expiration. Fluid balance must be maintained to stay healthy. There must be a balance between the amount of fluid taken in and the amount lost.

The amount of fluid taken in and the amount lost must be equal. If the fluid intake exceeds fluid output (the amount lost), body tissues swell with water. This is called *edema*. Edema is common in people with heart and kidney diseases. *Dehydration* is a decrease in the amount of water in the body tissues. It results when fluid output exceeds intake. Inadequate fluid intake, vomiting, diarrhea, bleeding, excessive sweating, and increased urine production are common causes of dehydration.

Normal requirements

An adult needs 1500 milliliters (ml) of water daily for survival. It requires 2000 to 2500 ml per day to maintain a normal fluid balance. The water requirement increases with higher outdoor temperatures, exercise, fever, and illness. Excessive fluid losses from the body also increase the water requirement. Minimum daily water requirements vary with age.

Special orders

The doctor may order the amount of fluid that a resident can have during a 24-hour period. This is done to maintain fluid balance. It may be necessary to force fluids. "Force fluids" involve having the individual consume an increased amount of fluid. When force fluids are ordered, records are kept of the amount taken in. The resident is given a variety of fluids that are allowed on the diet. They should be kept within the person's reach. You need to regularly offer fluids to residents who have force fluids orders but who are unable to feed themselves.

The doctor may write an order to restrict fluids. Fluids are restricted to a specific amount. Water is offered in small amounts and in small containers. The water pitcher is removed from the room or kept out of sight. Like the force fluids order, a sign is posted and accurate intake records are kept. The resident with restricted fluid intake needs to have frequent oral hygiene. Oral hygiene helps keep mucous membranes of the mouth moist.

Some residents are allowed nothing by mouth. This means the individual cannot eat or drink anything. NPO is the abbreviation for the Latin term "nils per os", which means nothing by mouth. Frequent oral hygiene is allowed as long as the resident does not swallow any fluid.

INTAKE AND OUTPUT RECORDS

The doctor or nurse may order that all of a resident's fluid intake and output be measured. The order involves keeping intake and output (I&O) records. The intake and output records are used to evaluate fluid balance and kidney function, and to determine and evaluate medical treatment. Intake and output records are also necessary when forcing fluids or restricting fluid intake.

Measurement of fluid intake involves measuring all liquid taken in by the resi-

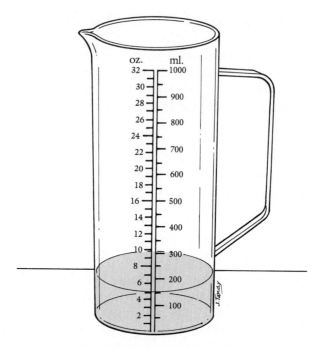

Fig. 13-2 A graduate calibrated in milliliters. It is filled to 150 ml. (*From Sorrentino SA: Mosby's textbook for nursing assistants, ed 3, St Louis, 1992, Mosby–Year Book.*)

dent through the mouth. Other fluids given in tube feedings are also measured. The obvious fluids are measured, such as water, milk, coffee, tea, juices, soups, and soft drinks. Soft and semisolid foods such as ice cream, sherbert, custard, pudding, creamed cereals, gelatin, and popsicles are also measured. Output includes urinary output, vomitus, diarrhea, and drainage from wounds.

Measuring intake and output

Intake and output are measured in milliliters (ml) or in cubic centimeters (cc). These are metric system measurements that are equal in amount. One ounce equals 30 ml. A pint equals about 500 ml. There are about 1000 ml in a quart. You need to know the fluid capacity of the bowls, dishes, cups, pitchers, glasses, and other containers used to serve fluids. Most health-care facilities provide conversion tables on the intake and output record for use in measuring intake.

A container called a *graduate* is used to measure fluids. You will use the graduate to measure leftover fluids, urine, vomitus, and drainage from suction. The graduate is similar to a measuring cup and shows calibrations for amounts. Some graduates are marked in ounces and in milliliters or cubic centimeters (Fig. 13-2). Plastic urinals and emesis basins are often calibrated.

An intake and output record is kept at the bedside. Whenever fluid is ingested or output measured, the amount is recorded in the appropriate column (Fig. 13-3). The amounts are totalled at the end of the shift. The nurse records the amount in the resident's record. The resident's intake and output are also communicated to the oncoming shift during the end-of-shift report. The nurse is responsible for recording any intake through tube feedings.

DAILY INTAKE AND OUTPUT RECORD
(Bedside record)

	Intake				Output		
11-7 Time	Oral	IV		Time	Urine	Emesis	Drainage

Total:_____   Total:_____

7-3 Time	Oral	IV		Time	Urine	Emesis	Drainage

Total:_____   Total:_____

3-11 Time	Oral	IV		Time	Urine	Emesis	Drainage

Total:_____   Total:_____

Water glass	= 150 ml	Milk carton	= 240 ml
Coffee pot	= 200 ml	Large paper cup	= 240 ml
Ice cream	= 60 ml	(like for eggnog,	
Coffee cup	= 120 ml	shakes, etc.)	
Soup bowl	= 180 ml	Jello per serving	= 120 ml

Fig. 13-3 An intake and output record. (*From Sorrentino SA:* Mosby's textbook for nursing assistants, *ed 3, St Louis, 1992, Mosby–Year Book.*)

The resident should receive an explanation about the purpose of measuring intake and output and how to participate in the process. Some residents may be taught how to measure and record their intake. Residents need to use a urinal, commode, bedpan, or specimen pan for urination. They need to be reminded not to put toilet tissue into the receptacle. Urine will be measured, so the resident should not urinate in the toilet.

To measure intake, pour liquid from the container to the graduate. Measure the amount in the graduate at eye level. Check the amount of the serving on the conversion list on the I&O record. Subtract the remaining liquid and total amounts. Record the amount and time in the intake column.

To measure output, pour the liquid into the graduate. Measure it at eye level. Record the amount and time on the I&O record. Clean equipment following the procedure.

ASSISTING THE INDIVIDUAL WITH FOODS AND FLUIDS

Weakness and illness can affect a person's appetite and ability to eat. Odors, the sight of unpleasant equipment, an uncomfortable position, the needs for oral hygiene, and the need to urinate are some factors that affect appetite. Nursing personnel can control these factors. You will often be responsible for preparing residents for meals.

Serving meal trays

Food is usually served in a dining room in a nursing facility. You will assist in serving meal trays after preparing residents for the meals. When serving meals on trays, it is important to serve the correct diet to each resident. The resident should be in a sitting position. The nurse aide needs to assist the resident as needed by opening boxes and packages (Fig. 13-4). Make sure the napkin and silverware are in the resident's reach.

Measure fluid intake as ordered. Note the amount and type of foods eaten by resident.

Feeding the resident

Some residents are unable to feed themselves. Weakness, paralysis, casts, and other physical limitations may make self-feeding impossible. These residents need to be fed. When feeding a resident you should be in a comfortable position. Many people say a prayer before eating. Providing time and privacy for a prayer conveys care and respect. You also need to consult with the resident about the order in which foods and fluids should be offered. A spoon is used when feeding residents because it is less likely to cause injury. When a resident is being fed, the spoon should only be one-third full (Fig. 13-5).

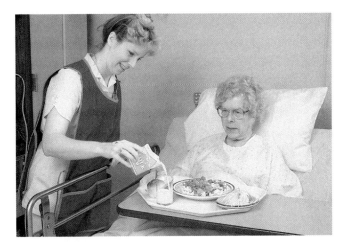

Fig. 13-4 The nurse aide opens containers for residents needing assistance. *(From Sorrentino SA:* Mosby's textbook for nursing assistants, *ed 3, St Louis, 1992, Mosby–Year Book.)*

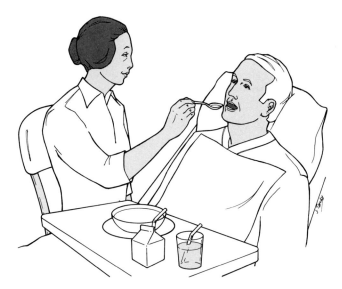

Fig. 13-5 A spoon is used to feed residents unable to feed themselves. The spoon should be no more than one-third full. *(From Sorrentino SA:* Mosby's textbook for nursing assistants, *ed 3, St Louis, 1992, Mosby–Year Book.)*

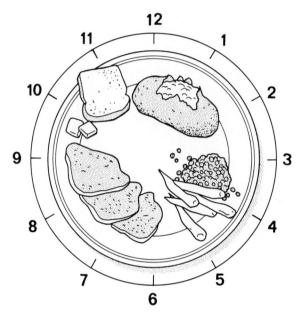

Fig. 13-6 The numbers on the face of a clock are used to help a blind person locate food. *(From Sorrentino SA:* Mosby's textbook for nursing assistants, *ed 3, St Louis, 1992, Mosby–Year Book.)*

Residents unable to feed themselves may feel anger, humiliation, and embarrassment at being dependent on others. Some may be depressed or resentful, or refuse to eat. Residents should be allowed to feed themselves as much as possible. You should provide residents with support and encouragement.

Many visually impaired people are keenly aware of food aromas. However, they need to know what foods and fluids are on the tray. When feeding a person who is visually impaired, you should always tell the person what you are offering. If the person does not need to be fed, you should identify the foods and their location on the tray. Use the numbers on a clock to identify the location of foods (Fig. 13-6).

Between-meal nourishments

Many therapeutic diets involve between-meal nourishments. Some of the commonly served nourishments are crackers, milk, juice, a milkshake, a piece of cake, wafers, a sandwich, gelatin, and custard. The resident should be served the nourishment as soon as it arrives on the nursing unit. The necessary eating utensils, a straw, and napkin need to be provided. The same considerations and procedures described for serving meal trays and feeding residents are followed.

Providing drinking water

Residents need to have fresh drinking water at periodic intervals. Fresh water is usually provided during the day and evening and whenever the pitcher is empty. Before passing out water, consult with the nurse about any special orders. Some residents may be NPO or on restricted fluids. You need to follow the rules of medical asepsis when passing out drinking water.

SUMMARY

The need for foods and fluids is basic for health and survival. A well-balanced diet contains foods from the four basic food groups. The diet provides the necessary amounts of proteins, carbohydrates, fats, vitamins, and minerals. Eating habits vary among individuals and are affected by a variety of factors, including religion and culture. When assisting a resident in meeting nutritional needs, you need to consider the factors that affect eating. Also try to make the meal as pleasant as possible for the individual.

Fluid balance is essential for health and life. The amount of fluid taken into the body must equal the amount lost. Fluid is lost through the urine, feces, skin, and lungs. You will assist doctors and nurses in evaluating a person's fluid balance by keeping accurate intake and output records when directed to do so.

Residents depend on nursing personnel to meet part or all of their food and fluid needs. They also need nourishments and fresh drinking water. Some residents need to be fed. Remember that meals provide opportunities for pleasure and socialization. The person should be in a comfortable sitting position for eating.

CHAPTER 14

Skin care

Objectives

Describe a decubitus ulcer
Identify sites where decubitus ulcers most often occur
List causes of decubiti
Describe nursing measures used to prevent decubiti

DECUBITUS ULCERS

Decubitus ulcers (decubiti) are areas where skin and underlying tissues are eroded due to a lack of blood flow (Fig. 14-1). They are also called *bedsores* and *pressure sores*. Decubiti occur most often in elderly, paralyzed, obese, or very thin and malnourished persons. The first sign of a decubitus ulcer is pale or white skin or a reddened area. The resident may complain of pain, burning, or tingling in the area. Some residents do not feel any abnormal sensations.

Sites

Decubitus ulcers occur over bony areas. The bony areas are called pressure points because they bear the weight of the body in a particular position. Pressure from body weight can reduce the blood supply to the area. Fig. 14-2 shows pressure points for the bed positions and the sitting position. In obese people, decubiti can develop in areas where skin is in contact with skin. Decubiti can develop between abdominal folds, the legs, the buttocks, and underneath the breasts.

Causes

Pressure and friction are common causes of skin breakdown and decubiti. Other contributing factors include breaks in the skin, poor circulation to an area, moisture, dry skin, and irritation by urine and feces. Individuals who are inactive or cannot move or change positions are at risk for decubiti.

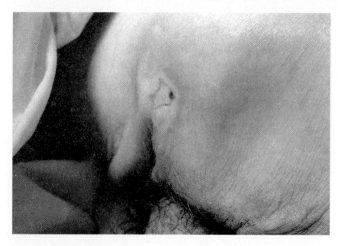

Fig. 14-1 A decubitus ulcer. (*From Sorrentino SA:* Mosby's textbook for nursing assistants, *ed 3, St Louis, 1992, Mosby–Year Book.*)

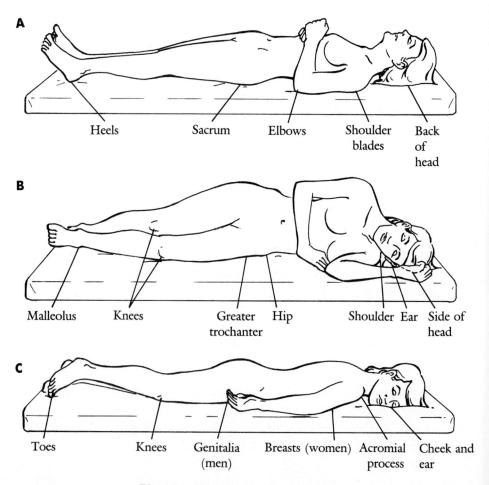

Fig. 14-2 For legend see opposite page.

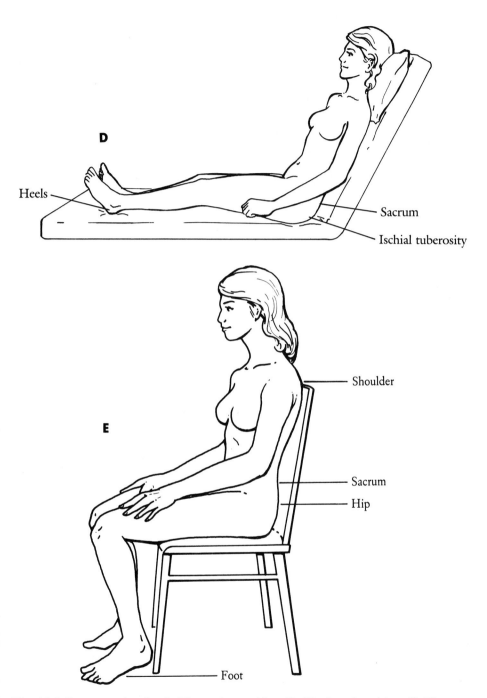

Fig. 14-2 Pressure points in: **A,** The supine position. **B,** The lateral position. **C,** The prone position. **D,** Fowler's position. **E,** Sitting position. *(From Sorrentino SA:* Mosby's textbook for nursing assistants, *ed 3, St Louis, 1992, Mosby–Year Book.)*

Prevention

Preventing decubitus ulcers is much easier than trying to heal them. Good nursing care, cleanliness, and skin care are essential. The following measures help prevent skin breakdown and decubiti.

1. Reposition the resident every 2 hours. Use pillows for support.
2. Provide good skin care. The skin must be clean and dry after bathing. Make sure the skin is free of urine, feces, and sweat.
3. Apply lotion to dry areas such as the hands, elbows, legs, ankles, and heels.
4. Give a back massage when repositioning the resident.
5. Keep linens clean, dry, and free of wrinkles.
6. Apply powder where skin touches skin.
7. Do not irritate the skin. Avoid scrubbing or vigorous rubbing when bathing or drying the resident.
8. Massage reddened or pale pressure points. Massage in a circular motion using lotion.
9. Use pillows and blankets to prevent skin from being in contact with skin and to reduce moisture and friction.
10. Immediately report any signs of skin breakdown or decubiti to the nurse.

Treatment

Treatment of decubitus ulcers is directed by the doctor. Drugs, treatments, and special equipment may be ordered to promote healing. The nurse and nursing care plan will tell you about a resident's treatment. Equipment used to treat and prevent decubiti are described in this section.

Sheepskin. Sheepskin (lamb's wool) is placed on the bottom sheet (Fig. 14-3) to protect skin from irritating bed linens. Friction is reduced between the skin and bottom sheet. Air circulates between the tufts to help keep the skin dry. Sheepskin comes in many sizes for use under the shoulders, buttocks, or heels.

Bed cradle. A bed cradle is a metal frame placed on the bed and over the resident. Top linens are brought over the cradle to prevent pressure on the legs and feet (Fig. 14-4). Top linens are tucked in at the bottom of the mattress and mitered. They are also tucked under both sides of the mattress to protect the resident from air drafts and chilling. The bed cradle is also called an *Anderson frame*.

Heel and elbow protectors. Heel and elbow protectors are made of foam rubber or sheepskin. They fit the shape of the heel or elbow (Fig. 14-5) and are secured in place with straps. Friction is prevented between the bed and the heel or elbow.

Flotation pad. Flotation pads or cushions (Fig. 14-6) are similar to water beds. They are made of a gel-like substance. The outer case is heavy plastic. They are used for chairs and wheelchairs. The pad is put into a pillowcase to prevent contact between the plastic case and the skin.

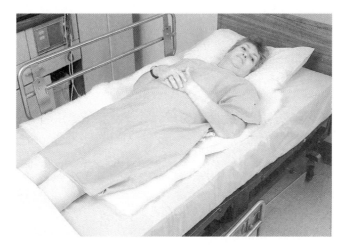

Fig. 14-3 Sheepskin. *(From Sorrentino SA:* Mosby's textbook for nursing assistants, *ed 3, St Louis, 1992, Mosby–Year Book.)*

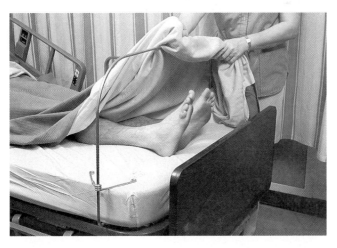

Fig. 14-4 A bed cradle. *(From Sorrentino SA:* Mosby's textbook for nursing assistants, *ed 3, St Louis, 1992, Mosby–Year Book.)*

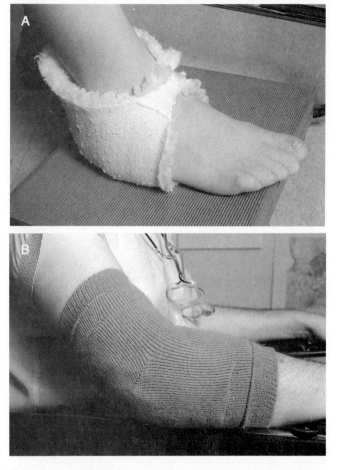

Fig. 14-5 A, Heel protector. **B,** Elbow protector. *(From Sorrentino SA:* Mosby's textbook for nursing assistants, *ed 3, St Louis, 1992, Mosby–Year Book.)*

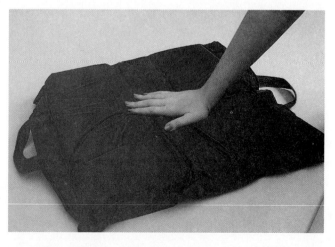

Fig. 14-6 Flotation cushion. *(From Sorrentino SA:* Mosby's textbook for nursing assistants, *ed 3, St Louis, 1992, Mosby–Year Book.)*

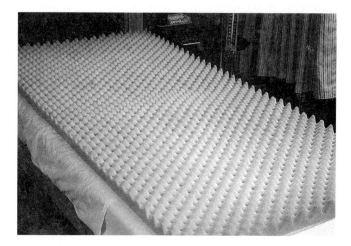

Fig. 14-7 Egg crate (foam) mattress. *(From Sorrentino SA:* Mosby's textbook for nursing assistants, *ed 3, St Louis, 1992, Mosby–Year Book.)*

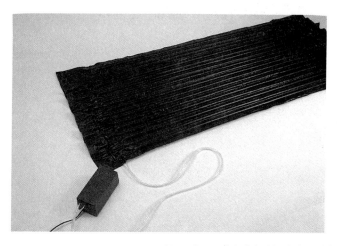

Fig. 14-8 The alternating pressure mattress. *(From Sorrentino SA:* Mosby's textbook for nursing assistants, *ed 3, St Louis, 1992, Mosby–Year Book.)*

The egg crate mattress. The egg crate (foam) mattress is a foam pad that looks like an egg carton (Fig. 14-7). Peaks in the mattress distribute the resident's weight more evenly. The egg crate mattress is placed on the regular mattress. Only a bottom sheet covers the egg crate mattress.

Water beds. Water beds are used in many facilities. The resident "floats" on top of the mattress. Body weight is distributed along the entire length of the body. Therefore, pressure on bony points is avoided.

Alternating pressure mattress. An alternating pressure mattress is electrically operated. It has vertical tube-like sections (Fig. 14-8). Every other section is inflated with air. The other sections are deflated. Every 3 to 5 minutes the sections deflate or inflate automatically. With this mattress, constant pressure on an area is avoided.

Only a bottom sheet is used with an alternating pressure mattress. Drawsheets and waterproof bed protectors are avoided. They add layers of material between the resident and air tubes. The air tubes should not be kinked. Pins are not used.

Clinitron bed. The Clinitron bed has a specially designed mattress. Air at a controlled temperature flows through the mattress. The resident "floats" on the mattress. Body weight is distributed evenly and pressure on body parts is minimal.

Guttman bed. The Guttman bed is used for position changes. The resident is rotated from right to left and to the supine position. The bed is useful for residents with spinal-cord injuries and those who are confined to bed.

SUMMARY

The resident's skin must be kept clean and intact. This promotes comfort and prevents infection. It's important for the nurse aide to observe for and report any skin breakdown. Proper positioning of the resident in the bed and chair and assisting in keeping the skin clean and dry will promote healthy, intact skin and prevent decubiti. Should they occur, follow the nurse's directions for treating them.

_____

CHAPTER 15

Transfers and Body Mechanics

Objectives

Explain the purpose and rules of testing good body mechanics

Identify guidelines for lifting and moving residents

Describe use of transfer (gait) belt in transferring or ambulating a resident

Explain how to use a mechanical lift safely

Identify the comfort and safety measures for using a stretcher to transport a resident

Nurse aides move residents often. A resident may be moved or turned in bed or transferred from the bed to a chair or wheelchair. During these and other activities, you need to use your body correctly to protect yourself from injury and to protect residents from the dangers of not being held or supported properly.

USING BODY MECHANICS

Using the body in an efficient and careful way is known as *body mechanics*. Body mechanics involves using good posture, balance, and the strongest and largest muscles of the body to perform work. Fatigue, muscle strain, and injury can result from improper use and positioning of the body during activity or rest. You need to be concerned with your body mechanics and that of your residents.

The major movable parts of the body are the head, trunk, arms, and legs. Posture, or body alignment, is the way body parts are aligned. Using good body alignment (posture) allows the body to move and function with strength and efficiency. Good alignment is necessary when standing, sitting, or lying down.

Base support is the area upon which an object rests. Feet provide the base of support for humans. A good base of support is needed to maintain balance. If you stand on one foot you will have difficulty balancing yourself or staying in the position for a long time. However, if you stand with your feet apart you will have a wider base of support. The wider base of support will make you feel more balanced

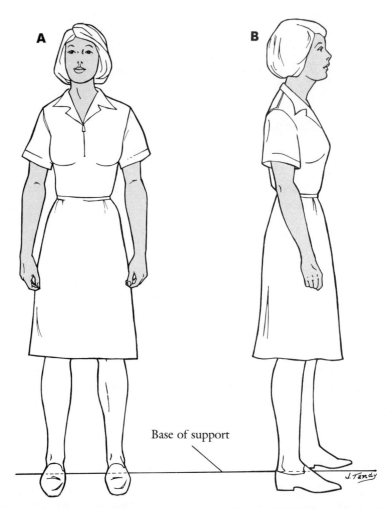

Fig. 15-1 A, Anterior view of adult in good body alignment with feet apart for a wide base of support. **B,** Lateral view of adult with good posture and alignment. *(From Sorrentino SA: Mosby's textbook for nursing assistants, ed 3, St Louis, 1992, Mosby–Year Book.)*

and stable. Therefore, the wider the base of support, the more balance and stability provided (Fig. 15-1).

The strongest and largest muscle groups are located in the shoulders, upper arms, hips, and thighs. These muscles should be used to lift and move heavy objects. If smaller and weaker muscle groups are used, strain and exertion is placed on them. This causes fatigue and injury (Fig. 15-2, *A*). You can use the strong muscles of your thighs and hips by bending your knees or squatting to lift a heavy object

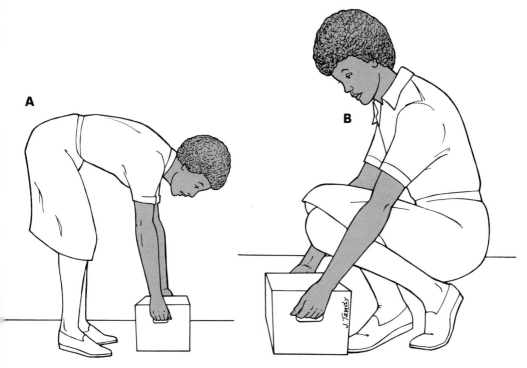

Fig. 15-2 A, Picking up a box with poor body mechanics. **B,** Picking up a box with good body mechanics. *(From Sorrentino SA:* Mosby's textbook for nursing assistants, *ed 3, St Louis, 1992, Mosby–Year Book.)*

(Fig. 15-2, *B*). You should avoid bending over from the waist when lifting. Bending from the waist involves the small muscles of the back. Holding objects close to the body and base of support involves using upper arm and shoulder muscles (Fig. 15-3). If the object is held away from the body, strain is exerted on the smaller muscles of the lower arms.

General rules

You should use good body mechanics in everyday activities. Most activities of daily living require good body mechanics. The following rules help you use good mechanics for safe and efficient functioning when lifting and moving residents and heavy objects.

1. Make sure your body is in good alignment and that you have a wide base of support.
2. Use the stronger and larger muscles of your body. These are located in the shoulders, upper arms, thighs, and hips.

3. Keep objects close to your body when lifting, moving, or carrying them.
4. Avoid unnecessary bending and reaching. If possible, have the height of the bed and overbed table level with your waist when giving care. You can adjust the bed and table to the proper height.
5. Face the direction in which you are working to prevent unnecessary twisting.
6. Push, slide, or pull heavy objects whenever possible rather than lifting them.
7. Use both of your hands and arms when lifting, moving, or carrying heavy objects.
8. Turn your whole body when you change the direction of your movement.
9. Work with smooth and even movements. Avoid sudden or jerky motions.
10. Get help from a co-worker to move heavy objects or residents whenever necessary.
11. Squat to lift heavy objects from the floor (see Fig. 15-2, *B*). Push against the strong muscles of your hips and thighs to raise yourself to a standing position.

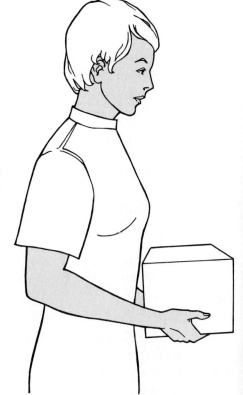

Fig. 15-3 Box being carried close to the body and base of support. (*From Sorrentino SA: Mosby's textbook for nursing assistants, ed 3, St Louis, 1992, Mosby–Year Book.*)

LIFTING AND MOVING RESIDENTS IN BED

Some residents can move and turn in bed by themselves. Others require the assistance of at least one person for position changes. Residents who are unconscious, paralyzed, on complete bed rest, in a cast, or weak from surgery or disease need assistance. Sometimes two or three people may be needed.

You should follow the rules of body mechanics when moving and lifting residents in bed. Residents should be protected from injury by being kept in good body alignment when being moved. The resident should be positioned in good body alignment after being moved.

Friction must be reduced to protect the resident's skin. Friction is the rubbing of one surface against another. When a resident is moved in bed, the resident's skin rubs against the sheet. This can result in scratching and skin injury. As a result, the resident is in danger of developing infection or decubitus ulcers. You can reduce friction when moving residents in bed by rolling or lifting instead of sliding them. A cotton drawsheet can be used as a turning sheet (lift or pull sheet) to move the resident in bed and thereby reduce friction. A nurse may suggest that the resident's skin or sheets be sprinkled with talcum powder or cornstarch to help reduce friction.

Other comfort and safety measures need to be considered before moving residents in bed. They are:

1. Consult the nurse for any limitations or restrictions in positioning or moving the resident. These may be ordered by the doctor or may be part of the resident's care plan.
2. Decide how the resident will be moved and how many helpers will be needed.
3. Get enough co-workers to help you before beginning the procedure.
4. Keep the resident covered and screened to protect the right to privacy.
5. Protect any tubes or drainage containers connected to the resident.

Raising the resident's head and shoulders

You may have to raise your resident's head and shoulders to tie the back of the gown, to turn or remove a pillow, or to give care. The resident's head and shoulders can be easily and safely raised by locking arms with the resident. Help may be needed if the resident is heavy or difficult to move (Fig. 15-4).

Moving the resident in bed

Many residents are able to have the head of their beds raised. When the head of the bed is raised, they often slide down toward the middle and foot of the bed. They will need to be moved up in bed to maintain good body alignment and comfort. You can usually move lightweight adults up in bed without help. Sometimes the resident is able to assist as in the following procedure.

To move a resident up in bed have the resident, if able, grasp the headboard of the bed and bend knees. The nurse aide has one arm under the resident's shoulder and other under the thighs. The resident is moved up in bed as the nurse aide's body weight is shifted from the rear to the front leg (Fig. 15-5 and 15-6).

Some residents require the assistance of two nurse aides. Nurses aides have locked arms under the resident. The resident's knees are flexed (Fig. 15-7).

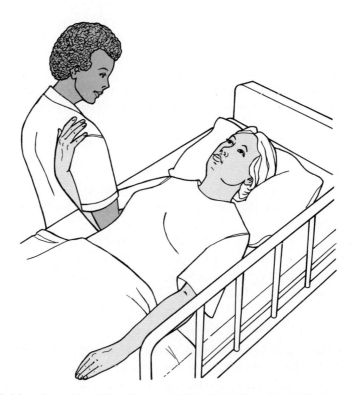

Fig. 15-4 Raising the resident's head and shoulders by locking arms with the resident. Resident near arm under the nurse aide's near arm and behind shoulder. (*From Sorrentino SA: Mosby's textbook for nursing assistants, ed 3, St Louis, 1992, Mosby–Year Book.*)

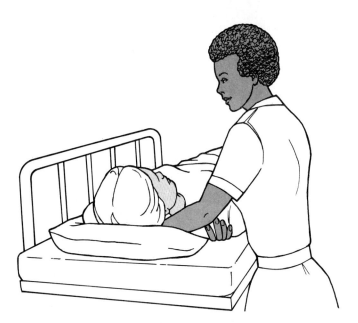

Fig. 15-5 Resident preparing to move up in bed. (*From Sorrentino SA:* Mosby's textbook for nursing assistants, *ed 3, St Louis, 1992, Mosby–Year Book.*)

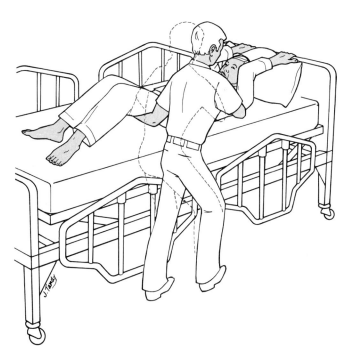

Fig. 15-6 Resident moved up in bed as nurse aide's body weight is shifted. (*From Sorrentino SA:* Mosby's textbook for nursing assistants, *ed 3, St Louis, 1992, Mosby–Year Book.*)

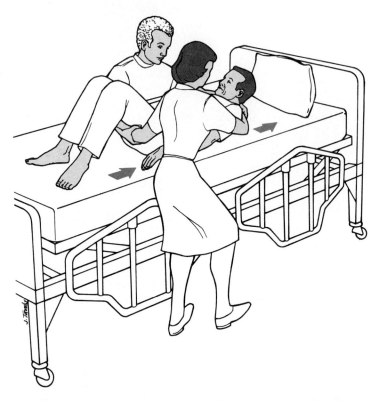

Fig. 15-7 Resident moved up in bed by two nurse aides. *(From Sorrentino SA:* Mosby's textbook for nursing assistants, *ed 3, St Louis, 1992, Mosby–Year Book.)*

Moving the resident up in bed using a turning (lift) sheet

With the help of a co-worker, you can easily and safely move a resident up in bed using a turning or lift sheet. Friction is reduced and the resident is lifted more evenly. A flat sheet folded in half or a drawsheet can be used for the turning sheet. The turning sheet is placed under the resident and should extend from the shoulders to above the knees. Certain residents should be moved up in bed with a turning sheet. These include those who are unconscious, paralyzed, or who have spinal-cord injuries (Figs. 15-8 and 15-9).

Moving a resident to the side of the bed

Residents are moved to the side of the bed when being repositioned and for certain procedures such as a bed bath. A resident lying in the middle of the bed needs to be moved to the side of the bed before being turned. Otherwise, after being turned, the resident will be lying on the side of the bed rather than in the middle. A resident should be lying in the middle of the bed to allow good body alignment.

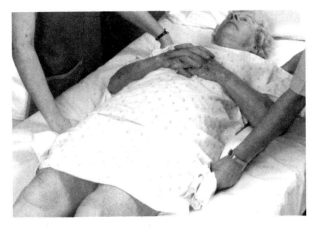

Fig. 15-8 Turning sheet is rolled up close to the resident. *(From Sorrentino SA:* Mosby's textbook for nursing assistants, *ed 3, St Louis, 1992, Mosby–Year Book.)*

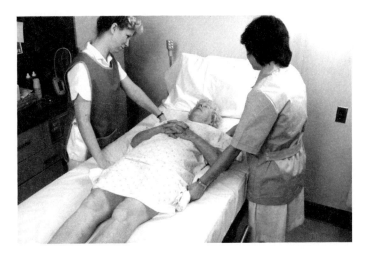

Fig. 15-9 Two nurse aides moving resident up in bed using a lift sheet. *(From Sorrentino SA:* Mosby's textbook for nursing assistants, *ed 3, St Louis, 1992, Mosby–Year Book.)*

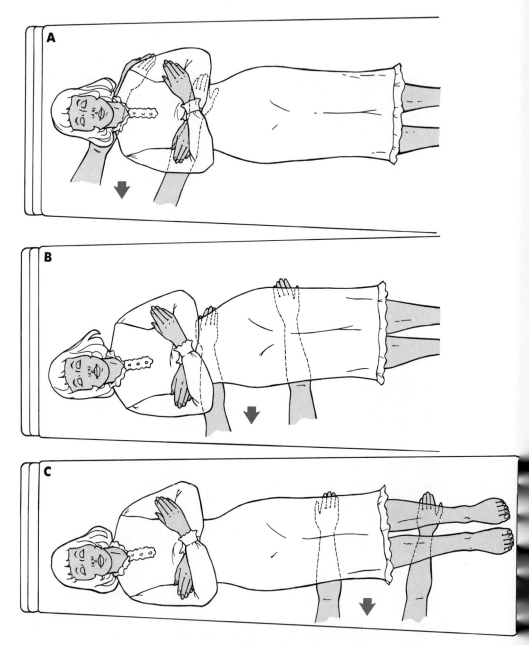

Fig. 15-10 A, Resident moved to side of bed in segments. Upper part of body moved first. **B,** Nurse aide has one arm under waist and other under thighs to move trunk. **C,** Residents legs and feet are moved to side of bed. *(From Sorrentino SA:* Mosby's textbook for nursing assistants, *ed 3, St Louis, 1992, Mosby–Year Book.)*

During certain procedures, such as a bed bath, you will have to reach over to the other side of the bed. Good body mechanics can be used if reaching is reduced and if the resident is close to you.

The resident should be in the back-lying position when being moved to the side of the bed. The procedure involves moving the resident in segments and can easily be done by one person. Do not use this procedure for residents with spinal-cord injuries or those recovering from spinal or back surgery (Fig. 15-10).

Turning residents

Residents have to be turned onto their sides to prevent complications from bedrest and to receive care. Certain nursing procedures require the side-lying position. Residents are turned toward or away from you. The direction depends on the resident's condition and the circumstances at the time.

To turn the resident toward you, have the resident cross his or her arms and legs. Place one hand on resident's far shoulder and the other on the far hip (Fig. 15-11).

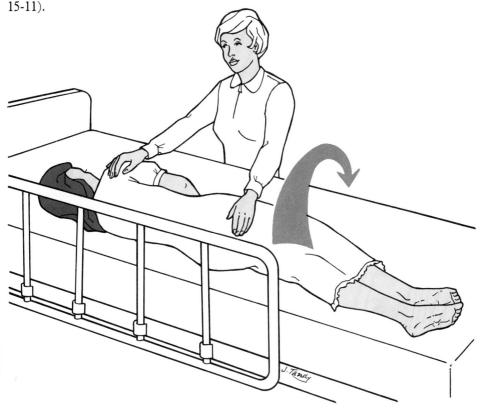

Fig. 15-11 Resident turned toward nurse aide. (*From Sorrentino SA:* Mosby's textbook for nursing assistants, *ed 3, St Louis, 1992, Mosby–Year Book.*)

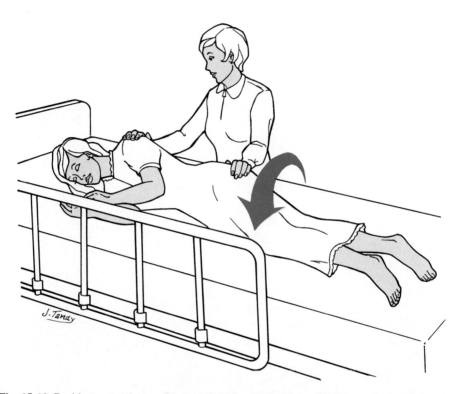

Fig. 15-12 Resident turned away from nurse aide. (*From Sorrentino SA:* Mosby's textbook for nursing assistants, *ed 3, St Louis, 1992, Mosby–Year Book.*)

To turn the resident away from you, assist the resident in crossing his or her arms and legs. Place one hand on resident's shoulder and the other on resident's buttock (Fig. 15-12).

Logrolling. Persons with spinal-cord injuries or those recovering from back surgery must keep their spines straight at all times. The resident must be rolled over in one motion. The back is kept in straight alignment when the resident is turned. Turning the resident as a unit in alignment with one motion is called *logrolling.* Two workers are needed to logroll a resident and three are needed if a resident is tall or heavy. Sometimes a turning sheet is useful for logrolling.

To logroll a resident, place a pillow between the resident's legs. His or her arms are crossed across the chest. The resident is on the far side of the bed. Nurse aides' hands are placed behind resident's shoulders and hips. The resident is turned toward the nurse aides without twisting. Place pillow supports against the back and under the head. Place a pillow or folded bath blanket between the resident's legs.

Sitting on the side of the bed (dangling)

Residents are helped to sit on the side of the bed, or dangle, for a variety of reasons. Some residents increase their activity in stages. They progress from bedrest to sitting on the side of the bed and then sitting in a chair. Walking about in the room and then in the hallway are the next steps. There are other reasons for a resident sitting on the side of the bed. These include preparing the resident to walk or to be transferred to a chair or wheelchair.

Two workers may be needed to help a resident sit on the side of the bed. If there is a problem with balance or coordination, the resident needs to be supported. The person should be returned to the lying position if fainting occurs. You need to make certain observations while the resident is dangling. The resident's pulse and respirations are taken and you need to observe for difficulty in breathing, pallor, or cyanosis (blue skin). Also note any complaints of dizziness or lightheadedness.

To dangle the resident or bring to a sitting position, the nurse aide should use good body mechanics and assist the resident in turning toward the nurse aide. Place one hand behind the resident's shoulder and the other hand behind the resident's knee. Bring the resident to a sitting position with his or her feet on the floor or a stool.

TRANSFERRING RESIDENTS

Residents need to be moved from their beds to chairs, wheelchairs, or stretchers. Some need only minimal assistance in transferring. Semihelpless residents require the assistance of at least one person. A helpless resident needs to be transferred by at least two or three people. The general rules of body mechanics and the safety and comfort considerations described for lifting and moving residents also apply when transferring residents. The room should be arranged to provide enough space for a safe transfer. The chair, wheelchair, or stretcher must be placed correctly for safe and efficient transfer.

A transfer belt is useful when transferring a semihelpless or helpless resident. The belt is applied around the resident's waist. You can grasp the belt to hold onto the resident during the transfer. The belt is also called a *gait belt* and is used when walking with a resident (Fig. 15-13).

Have the chair or commode at an angle at bedside. Bring the resident to a sitting position, apply shoes (these may be applied while resident is in the supine position). Apply the transfer belt. Grasp the transfer belt at the sides. Brace your knees against the resident's knees for support. Ask the resident to place his or her hands on your shoulders. Using good body mechanics, bring the resident to a standing position. Continue to block the resident's knees and support him or her with the transfer belt. Turn the resident to the chair. Have the resident place his or her hands on the wheelchair or commode arms (Figs. 15-14, 15-15, 15-16 and 15-17). Slowly bend your knees, keep your back straight, and lower the resident into the chair or commode.

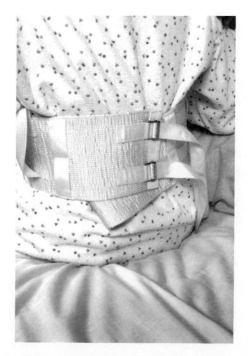

Fig. 15-13 Transfer belt. (*From Sorrentino SA:* Mosby's textbook for nursing assistants, *ed 3, St Louis, 1992, Mosby–Year Book.*)

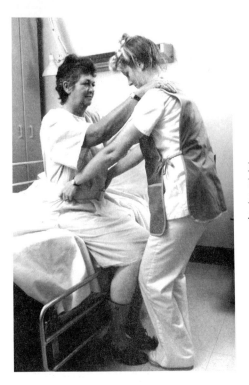

Fig. 15-14 Transferring a resident while blocking the knees. (*From Sorrentino SA:* Mosby's textbook for nursing assistants, *ed 3, St Louis, 1992, Mosby–Year Book.*)

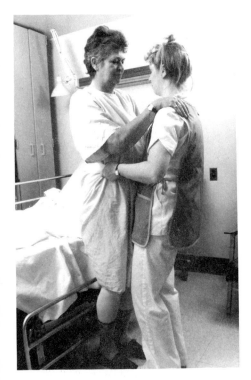

Fig. 15-15 Transferring a resident bringing resident to a standing position. (*From Sorrentino SA:* Mosby's textbook for nursing assistants, *ed 3, St Louis, 1992, Mosby–Year Book.*)

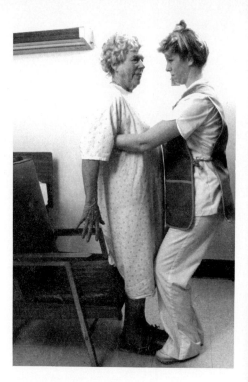

Fig. 15-16 Transferring a resident. Resident is supported as she grasps arm of chair. The resident's calves are against the chair. *(From Sorrentino SA:* Mosby's textbook for nursing assistants, *ed 3, St Louis, 1992, Mosby–Year Book.)*

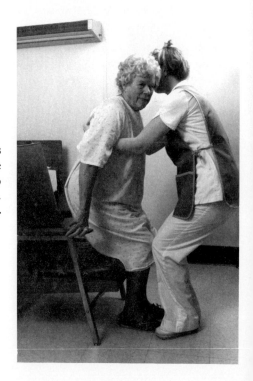

Fig. 15-17 Resident holds armrests, leans forward, and bends elbows and knees while being lowered into chair. *(From Sorrentino SA:* Mosby's textbook for nursing assistants, *ed 3, St Louis, 1992, Mosby–Year Book.)*

Transferring a patient to a chair or wheelchair

Safety is a major consideration when transferring a resident to a chair or wheelchair. The resident needs to be protected from falling. Street shoes should be worn to prevent the resident from sliding or slipping on the floor. In addition, the chair or wheelchair must be sturdy enough to support the resident's weight. The number of assistants required for a transfer will depend on the resident's physical capabilities, condition, and size. The resident should be encouraged to help in the transfer whenever possible to help increase muscle strength.

Most wheelchairs or bedside chairs have vinyl seats and backs. The vinyl retains body heat, causing the resident to become warmer and perspire more. You can cover the back and seat with a folded bath blanket, a pillow, or wheelchair cushion on the seat. This will increase the resident's comfort when sitting in the chair.

You need to know which side of the resident's body is the strong side. You should help the resident out of bed on his or her strong side. If the resident's left side is weak and the right side strong, the resident should get out of bed on the right side.

When transferring to a chair or wheelchair, the strong side will move first and pull the weaker side along. Transferring a resident from the weak side results in an awkward and unsafe transfer.

The nurse may request that the resident's pulse be taken before and after the transfer. The resident may not have been out of bed before or may tire with even a little exertion. The pulse rate provides some information about how the activity was tolerated. You should also observe and report if the resident tires easily, complains of weakness or being lightheaded, experiences pain or discomfort, or has difficulty in breathing (dyspnea). Also report the amount of help needed and how the resident participated in the transfer.

Mechanical lifts

A mechanical lift is used to transfer helpless residents. The resident may be transferred from a bed to a chair, stretcher, bathtub, toilet, whirlpool, or car. Before using the lift you need to make sure it is functioning. You need to compare the resident's weight and weight limit of the lift. The lift must not be used for a resident whose weight exceeds its capacity.

Many facilities have policies stating that at least two people are needed to transfer a resident with a mechanical lift. Be sure you are familiar with the policy of your facility regarding mechanical lifts.

To perform this procedure:

1. Provide for safety and privacy.
2. Position sling under the resident. Lower edge should be under the resident's knees.
3. Release valve of mechanical lift should be in closed position.

4. Position lift over resident and widen the base of support.
5. Attach sling to lift so that hooks are turned away from the resident's body.
6. Attach sling to swivel bar.
7. Raise lift until sling and resident clear the bed.
8. Support the resident's legs and move lift away from the bed.
9. Guide resident into the chair.

Moving the resident to a stretcher

Stretchers are used to transfer residents who are helpless and unable to sit up, those who must remain in a lying position, and residents who are ill.

The stretcher should be covered with a folded flat sheet or bath blanket. A pillow and a sufficient number of blankets should be available. To increase the resident's comfort, the head of the stretcher can be raised to a sitting or semisitting position.

The safety straps are applied after the resident is transferred to the stretcher. The side rails of the stretcher are kept up when transporting the resident. The resident should be moved feet first so the helper at the head of the stretcher can observe the resident. A resident on a stretcher should never be left unattended.

Using a drawsheet. A drawsheet can be used to transfer a patient from the bed to a stretcher. At least three workers are needed to perform the transfer safely. Remember to keep the resident in good body alignment and to use good body mechanics.

SUMMARY

Good body mechanics must be used at all times when lifting, moving, and transferring residents to protect yourself and the resident from injury. You need to keep yourself and the resident in good body alignment to promote comfort and physical well-being.

You have learned several ways to move, lift, and transfer residents in bed. Resident comfort and safety must always be considered during these activities. Also be sure to protect the resident's right to privacy and safety from falling. The resident should be encouraged to participate in transfers to the extent possible.

You may need to change some life-long habits in relation to your posture and the way you move your body. As you practice using good body mechanics, you will find that you feel better and are able to do more work with greater efficiency.

CHAPTER 16

Mental Health and Social Service Needs

Objectives

Identify Maslow's Hiearchy of Needs
Define mental health
Describe mental illness
Explain how culture and religion affect the resident's behavior during illness
Identify the developmental tasks of the elderly
Describe sexuality as it relates to the elderly
Discuss the effects of injury and illness on sexuality
Identify how to manage a sexually aggressive resident
Explain the importance of family and friends to the resident's psychological or emotional well-being

In the busy world of health care it is easy to forget that the resident in a nursing facility has been an active member of a community. Things are now done to and for the resident. The resident usually has to adjust to different patterns of what to eat and when to eat, sleep, bathe, have visitors, sit in a chair, walk, and use the bathroom. They often feel that nurses, nurse aides, and other health workers treat them as objects rather than people. Most residents receive care for physical problems. However, to effectively care for residents you must be aware of the whole person.

The whole person consists of physical, social, psychological, and spiritual parts. The parts are woven together and cannot be separated (Fig. 16-1). Each part relates to and depends upon the others.

As a social being, a person speaks and communicates with others. Physically, the brain, mouth, tongue, lips, and throat structures must function for speech. Communication is also highly psychological because it involves the thinking and reasoning abilities of the mind. To consider only the physical part is to ignore the resident's ability to think, make decisions, and interact with others. It also ignores the fact that the resident is a living person with experiences, joys, sorrows, and needs.

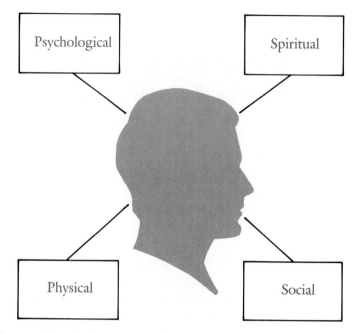

Fig. 16-1 A person is a physical, psychological, social, and spiritual being. The parts overlap and cannot be separated. (*From Sorrentino SA:* Mosby's textbook for nursing assistants, *ed 3, St Louis, 1992, Mosby–Year Book.*)

NEEDS

A *need* is that which is necessary or desirable for maintaining life and mental well-being. According to Abraham Maslow, a famous psychologist, certain basic needs must be met if a person is to survive and function. These needs are arranged in order of importance. The lower level needs must be met before the higher level. These basic needs, from the lowest level to the highest, are: physiologic or physical needs, the need for safety and security, the need for love and belonging, esteem needs, and the need for self-actualization (Fig. 16-2). People normally meet their own needs every day. When they are unable to meet their basic needs, it is usually because of disease, illness, or injury. When ill, they usually seek help from doctors, nurses, and other health team members.

Physiological needs

Humans share certain physiological (physical) needs with other forms of life, such as animals, fish, and plants. Physical needs necessary for life are oxygen, food, water, elimination, and rest. These needs are the most important for survival. They must be met before higher level needs.

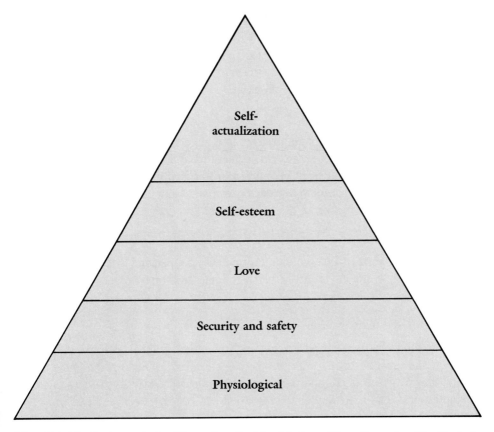

Fig. 16-2 The basic needs for life as described by Maslow. *(From Sorrentino SA:* Mosby's textbook for nursing assistants, *ed 3, St Louis, 1992, Mosby–Year Book.)*

An individual will die within minutes without oxygen. People can survive longer without food or water, but will begin to feel weak and ill within a few hours. If the kidneys or intestines are not functioning normally, poisonous wastes build up in the bloodstream. If the problem is not corrected, the person will die. Without enough rest and sleep an individual will become exhausted.

You will assist nurses to help residents meet their physical needs, such as thirst, hunger, and sleep.

The need for safety and security

Safety and security needs relate to the need for shelter, clothing, and protection from harm or danger. Problems from inadequate shelter or clothing are often dealt with by health workers.

Many people feel that certain medical and nursing procedures are harmful or dangerous. This is not surprising since many procedures involve frightening equipment, require entering the body, and cause pain or discomfort. Residents feel safer and more secure if they know why a procedure needs to be done, how it will be performed, and the sensations they can expect to feel.

The need for love and belonging

The need for love and belonging relates to love, closeness, affection, belonging, and meaningful relationships with others. There have been many cases where residents have had slow recoveries or have given up their will to live because of lack of love and belonging. The resident's need for love and belonging can be met by family, friends, and health workers.

The need for esteem

Esteem is the worth, value, or opinion one has of a person. Esteem needs relate to thinking well of one's self and of being thought well of by others. People often lack esteem when ill or injured.

The need for self-actualization

Self-actualization means experiencing one's potential. It involves learning, understanding, and creating to the limit of a person's capacity. This is the highest need. Rarely, if ever, is this need totally met. Most people constantly try to learn and understand more. The need for self-actualization can be postponed and life will continue.

Mental health

A mentally healthy person is one whose needs are met, who is coping adequately, and who has feelings of self-worth. Physical and emotional illness can occur when coping with stress is not adequate and needs go unmet. The nurse aide can promote mental health by assisting residents to meet their needs as described.

CULTURE AND RELIGION

Culture is defined as values, beliefs, habits, likes, dislikes, customs, and characteristics of a group of people that are passed from one generation to the next. The resident's culture influences health beliefs and practices. Culture also influences behavior during illness.

You will care for people from different cultural backgrounds. Besides caring for Americans of various national backgrounds, you may care for people from other cultures and countries. These people have family practices, food preferences, hygiene habits, and clothing styles that are different from yours. The person may also speak and understand a foreign language. Some cultural groups have beliefs about the causes and cures of illnesses. They may perform certain rituals aimed at ridding the body of disease.

Religion relates to spiritual beliefs, needs, and practices. Like culture, an individual's religion influences health and illness practices. Religions have beliefs and practices relating to diet, healing, days of worship, birth, and death.

Most Americans are of the Jewish, Protestant, or Roman Catholic faiths. Many people find religion to be a source of comfort and strength during illness. They may wish to observe religious practices and may appreciate a visit from their spiritual leader or adviser (such as a rabbi, preacher, or priest). If a resident requests such a visit, promptly report the request to the nurse.

Make sure the resident's room is neat and orderly, and place a chair by the bed for the visitor's use. Allow privacy during the visit.

You must show respect and accept the resident's cultural and religious background. When you meet people from other cultures or religions, take advantage of the chance to learn about their beliefs and practices. This will help you understand your resident and give better care.

Individuals may not follow all beliefs and practices of a culture or religion. Remember, each person is unique. Do not judge residents or impose your beliefs on them.

ILLNESS

If people had a choice between staying healthy or becoming ill, health would be selected. Unfortunately, people become ill and injured. Besides physical problems caused by illness, the sick person experiences psychological and social effects.

The resident may be unable to perform normal daily activities. Daily activities bring personal satisfaction, self-worth, and contact with others. Most people feel frustrated and angry when unable to perform them. These feelings may become even greater if others must perform these activities for the resident.

Sick people have many fears and anxieties. There is fear of death, disability, chronic illness, and loss of function.

DEVELOPMENTAL TASKS

Persons in late adulthood (65 years and older) experience many physical, psychological, and social changes. This group is referred to as the elderly. Developmental tasks of the elderly are:

1. Adjusting to decreased physical strength and loss of health.
2. Adjusting to retirement and reduced income.
3. Developing new friends and relationships.
4. Preparing for death.

It's important that nurse aides be familiar with these changes and provide residents with understanding and respect.

SEXUALITY AND THE ELDERLY

In the past, residents were viewed as having only physical problems. Therefore, physical needs were the first and often the only concern. Little attention was given to psychological or social needs. The needs of love and belonging, esteem, and self-actualization were overlooked. Now attention is given to the total person. Physical, psychological, social, and spiritual aspects of the person are considered.

Another part of the person involves the physical, psychological, social, and the spiritual. That part is sexuality. The effect of illness and injury on a resident's sexuality is now recognized.

Sex and sexuality are different. Sex is the physical activities involving the reproductive organs. The activities are done for pleasure or to have children. *Sexuality* involves the whole personality and the body. A resident's attitudes and feelings are involved. Besides physical and psychological factors, sexuality is influenced by social, cultural, and spiritual factors. The way a person behaves, thinks, dresses, and responds to others is related to his or her sexuality.

Many people think that sex, love, and intimacy are only for the young. They believe that older people are not supposed to need these things. There is also the false idea that older people are not capable of sexual activities. Fortunately, these ideas are untrue. Sexual relationships are psychologically and physically important to the elderly. Love, affection, and intimacy are needed throughout life.

Effects of injury and illness

Sexuality and sex involve the mind and body. Injury and illness can affect the way the body works. Many illnesses, injuries, and surgeries cause changes in the nervous, circulatory, and reproductive systems. If one or more of these systems are affected, the resident may experience changes in sexual functioning or ability. Most chronic illnesses affect the resident's sexual functioning.

You will care for residents with disorders that can affect sexual functioning. Changes in sexual functioning have a great impact. Fear, anger, worry, and depression often occur. These are evident in the resident's behavior and comments. You need to understand that the resident's feelings are normal and expected.

Meeting the resident's sexual needs

Sexuality is part of the total person. Illness, injury, or aging does not mean that sexuality is unimportant. Sexual activity does not always mean intercourse. It may be expressed in other ways. Nursing personnel used to discourage any form of sexual expression, especially among the elderly. Hand holding was okay, but two people were not to get any closer! The importance of sexuality in health and illness is now recognized. The nursing team has an important role in allowing residents to meet their sexual needs. The following measures are appreciated by residents. They are carried out in cooperation with the nurse supervising your work.

1. Allow the person to practice grooming routines.
2. Allow the person personal choices about clothing selection.
3. Avoid exposing the resident. Provide for the resident's privacy.
4. Accept the resident's sexual relationships. Do not make judgments or gossip about these relationships.
5. Allow privacy. Some facilities have "do not disturb" signs for doors. Let the resident and partner know how much time they can expect to have alone. Consideration must be given to a roommate. The curtain between the two beds provides little privacy. Privacy can be arranged when the roommate is out of the room. If the roommate cannot leave, other areas on the nursing unit can be found for privacy.
6. Allow couples in nursing facilities to share a room. (This is now an OBRA requirement.) They should be allowed to share the same bed if their conditions permit.
7. Allow single persons to develop new relationships. Death and divorce result in loss of sexual partners. A widowed or divorced resident may develop a relationship with another resident.

The sexually aggressive resident

Some residents try to have their sexual needs met by flirting or making sexual advances toward health workers. If this happens, health workers usually become angry or embarrassed. These reactions are normal. Often there are reasons for the resident's behavior. Understanding the resident's behavior may help you deal with the situation.

Illness, injury, surgery, or aging may threaten the male's sense of manhood. He may try to reassure or prove to himself that he is still attractive and capable of performing sexually. He may do so by behaving sexually toward health workers.

Some sexually aggressive behaviors are due to confusion or disorientation. Nervous system disorders, medications, fever, dementia, and poor vision are common causes of confusion and disorientation. The resident may actually confuse a worker with his or her sexual partner, or the resident may be unable to control behavior because of changes in mental function. The person would normally be able to control urges toward a worker. However, changes in the brain can make control difficult. Sexual behavior in these situations is usually innocent on the resident's part.

Some residents do touch staff inappropriately. Their purpose is sexual. However, sometimes touch is the only way to get the nurse aide's attention.

Sexual advances may be intentional. You need to deal with this in a professional manner. However, there is no ideal way to deal with the advances. The following suggestions may be helpful.

1. Discuss the situation with the nurse. The nurse can help you deal with or understand the resident's behavior.
2. Ask the resident not to touch you in places where you were touched.
3. Explain to the resident that you have no intention of doing what he or she suggests.
4. Explain to the resident that his or her behavior makes you uncomfortable. Then politely ask the resident not to act in that way.
5. Allow privacy if the resident becomes sexually aroused. Provide for safety (for example, raise side rails and place the signal light within reach) and tell the person when you will return.

THE RESIDENT'S FAMILY AND VISITORS

Family, relatives, and friends can help meet the resident's needs for safety and security, love and belonging, and esteem. They can offer support and comfort and lessen feelings of loneliness. Some also assist in the resident's care. They may help with such things as meals, bathing, and brushing or combing hair.

The resident should be allowed to visit with family and friends in private and without unnecessary interruptions. Sometimes care must be given to residents when visitors are present. You should politely ask them to step out of the room and show them where they can wait comfortably. Do not expose the resident in front of visitors. Promptly notify the visitors when they can return to the room.

Family and visitors must be treated with courtesy and respect. They need the support and understanding of the nursing team. However, to protect the resident's privacy, do not discuss the resident's condition with them. Refer questions to the nurse responsible for the resident's care.

Residents who are terminally ill are usually allowed to have family members present at the bedside constantly. Know the visiting policies of your facility and the special considerations allowed.

Sometimes a family member or friend can have a negative effect on the resident. If the resident becomes upset or is becoming tired because of a visitor, report your observations to the nurse. The nurse can then speak with the visitor about the resident's needs.

SUMMARY

People are physical, psychological, spiritual, and social humans. They have certain basic needs necessary for life: physical needs, the need for safety and security, love and belongings, esteem, and self-actualization. When the residents in a nursing facility cannot meet their needs, they require the help of health-care workers.

Culture and religion influence behavior of residents, especially when ill. Being sick affects a person physically, psychologically, and socially.

The elderly go through many life changes. The nurse aide needs to understand the life changes and cultural practices of residents to provide effective care.

Sexuality is part of the total person. People that are ill, injured, or older still need love, affection, and closeness with other people. Health workers should promote, not discourage, the resident's sexual expression.

Family and friends of the resident provide support and love. It is important that the nurse aide be respectful of visitors.

SUMMARY

CHAPTER 17

Care of Cognitively Impaired Residents

Objectives

Explain chronic brain syndrome

Describe the care required by persons with chronic brain syndrome

Describe Alzheimer's disease

Describe the signs, symptoms, and behaviors of Alzheimer's disease

Explain the care required by persons with Alzheimer's disease

Describe the effects of Alzheimer's disease on the family

Changes in the brain occur with aging. Certain diseases can also cause changes in the brain. These changes can affect the resident's intellectual functioning. Intellectual functioning relates to memory, thinking, reasoning, ability to understand, judgment, and behavior. *Dementia* is the term used to describe mental disorders caused by changes in the brain. Dementias are chronic. There is no cure and the disease becomes progressively worse.

CHRONIC BRAIN SYNDROME

Chronic brain syndrome affects the ability to think and understand. Changes in brain cells occur. The changes may be due to decreased blood flow, atrophy, chemicals, infections, poor nutrition, or the aging process.

Signs and symptoms of chronic brain syndrome develop slowly. They may go unnoticed for a long time. There may be memory loss. Also, the person may be unable to remember something that happened yesterday or a few minutes ago, while events of the long ago past are remembered. Disorientation occurs. The person may not know the date, time, or place. People may not be recognized or the resident may

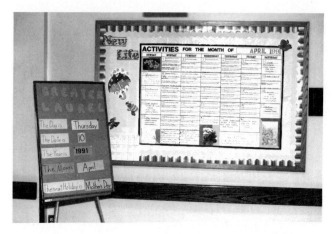

Fig. 17-1 A reality orientation board is used as part of reality orientation. *(From Sorrentino SA:* Mosby's textbook for nursing assistants, *ed 3, St Louis, 1992, Mosby–Year Book.)*

not remember names. The ability to concentrate decreases. The resident may be unable to follow simple instructions. Judgement is poor. The resident may not recognize harmful situations. Attention to personal hygiene decreases.

Reality orientation (promoting awareness of person, time, and place) is important for residents with chronic brain syndrome (Fig. 17-1). The resident may be partially or totally dependent on others for basic needs. Supervision and assistance in activities of daily living are needed. The resident must also be protected from injury.

ALZHEIMER'S DISEASE

Alzheimer's disease is a brain disease. Brain cells that control intellectual functioning are damaged. It occurs in men and women. Though it is more common in the elderly, it also occurs in younger people. Some people in their 40s and 50s have Alzheimer's disease. The cause is unknown.

Stages of Alzheimer's disease

Three stages of Alzheimer's disease have been described. Signs and symptoms become more severe with each stage. The disease ends in death. The stages are described in the box on p. 245.

Wandering, sundowning, hallucinations, and delusions also occur. Residents with Alzheimer's disease are disoriented to people, time, and place. They may wander from home and not be able to find their way back. They may be with caregivers one minute and gone the next. Remember, residents with Alzheimer's disease have poor judgment and cannot tell what is safe or dangerous. They are in danger of ac-

STAGES OF ALZHEIMER'S DISEASE

Stage 1
Memory loss and forgetfulness, forgets recent events
Poor judgment, bad decisions
Disoriented to time
Lack of spontaneity—less outgoing or interested in things
Blames others for mistakes, forgetfulness, and other problems
Moodiness

Stage 2
Restlessness, which often increases during the evening hours
Sleep disturbances
Memory loss increases—may not recognize family and friends
Dulled senses—cannot tell the difference between hot and cold,
  cannot recognize dangers
Bowel and bladder incontinence
Needs assistance with activities of daily living—problems with
  bathing, feeding, and dressing self, afraid of bathing, will not
  change clothes
Loses impulse control—may use foul language, have poor table
  manners, sexually aggressive, or rude
Movement and gait disturbances—walks slowly, has a shuffling gait
Communication problems—cannot follow directions; problems with
  reading, writing, and math; speaks in short sentences or just
  words; statements may not make sense
Repeats motions and statements—may move things back and forth
  constantly; may say the same thing over and over again
Agitation—behavior may become violent

Stage 3
Cannot communicate—may groan, grunt, or scream
Does not recognize self or family members
Totally dependent on others for all activities of daily living
Disoriented to person, time, and place
Totally incontinent of urine and feces
Cannot swallow—choking and aspiration are risks
Sleep disturbances increase
Becomes bed bound—cannot sit or walk
Coma
Death

cidents. A person may walk into traffic or into a river or lake. If not properly dressed, there is the risk of exposure in cold climates.

Sundowning occurs in the late afternoon and evening hours. As daylight ends and darkness occurs, confusion, restlessness, and other symptoms increase. The resident's behavior is worse at night after the sun goes down. Sundowning may relate to being tired or hungry. Inadequate light may cause the resident to see things that are not there. Like children, residents with Alzheimer's disease may be afraid of the dark.

Senses are dulled. The resident may see, hear, or feel things that are not real. A *hallucination* is seeing, hearing, or feeling something that is not really there. People may see animals, insects, or people that are not present. Some hear voices. They may feel bugs crawling on their bodies or feel that they are being touched.

Delusions are false beliefs. People with Alzheimer's disease have thought that they were the Lord, movie stars, or some other person. Some believe they are in jail, are going to be murdered, or are being attacked. A resident may believe that the caregiver is actually someone else. Many other false beliefs can occur.

Care of the person with Alzheimer's disease

Alzheimer's disease is frustrating to the resident, family, and caregivers. Usually the person is cared for at home until symptoms become severe. Care in a nursing facility is often required. The resident may develop other illnesses and need hospital care. The resident and the family needs your support and understanding.

You must remember that residents with Alzheimer's disease do not choose to be forgetful, incontinent, agitated, or rude. They do not choose to have all of the other behaviors, signs, and symptoms of the disease. They have no control over what is happening to them. The disease causes the behaviors. When a resident does something that a healthy person would not do, remember that the disease is responsible, not the resident.

Care of residents with Alzheimer's disease is described in the box on pp. 247-248. Such measures will probably be part of the resident's care plan.

The family

The family of the resident with Alzheimer's disease has special needs. Caring for the loved one can be exhausting. They need much support and encouragement. Many join Alzheimer's disease support groups. These groups are sponsored by hospitals, nursing facilities, and the Alzheimer's Association. The Alzheimer's Association has chapters in cities and towns throughout the country. Support groups offer encouragement, advice, and ideas about care. People in similar situations share their feelings, anger, frustration, and other emotions.

The family often feels helpless. No matter what is done for the loved one, the resident only gets worse. Much time, money, energy, and emotion are required to

CARE OF THE PERSON WITH ALZHEIMER'S DISEASE

Safety

- Remove sharp and breakable objects from the environment. This includes knives, scissors, glass, dishes, and razors.
- Provide plastic eating and drinking utensils. This prevents possible breakage and cuts.
- Place safety plugs in electrical outlets.
- Keep cords and electrical equipment out of reach.
- Childproof caps should be on medicine containers and household cleaners.
- Store household cleaners and medicines in locked storage areas.
- Practice safety measures to prevent falls.
- Practice safety measures to prevent burns.
- Practice safety measures to prevent poisoning.

Wandering

- Make sure doors and windows are securely locked.
- Make sure door alarms are turned on. The alarm goes off when the door is opened. These are common in nursing facilities.
- Make sure the resident wears an ID bracelet at all times.
- Exercise the resident as ordered. Adequate exercise often reduces wandering.

Wandering—cont'd

- Do not restrain the resident. Restraints require a doctor's order. They also tend to increase confusion and disorientation.
- Do not argue with the resident who wants to leave. Remember, the resident does not understand what you are saying.
- Go with the resident who insists on going outside. Make sure he or she is properly dressed. Guide the resident inside after a few minutes.
- Let the resident wander in enclosed areas if provided. Many nursing facilities have enclosed areas where residents can walk about. These areas provide a safe place for the resident to wander.

Sundowning

- Provide a calm, quiet environment late in the day. Treatments and activities should be done early in the day.
- Do not restrain the resident.
- Encourage exercise and activity early in the day.
- Make sure the resident has eaten. Hunger can increase the resident's restlessness.
- Promote urinary and bowel elimination. A full bladder or constipation can increase restlessness.

Continued.

CARE OF THE PERSON WITH ALZHEIMER'S DISEASE—CONT'D

Sundowning—cont'd

- Do not try to reason with the resident. Remember, he or she cannot understand what you are saying.
- Do not ask the resident to tell you what is bothering him or her. The resident's ability to communicate is impaired. He or she does not understand what you are asking. Nor can the resident think and speak clearly.

Hallucinations and delusions

- Do not argue with the resident. He or she does not understand what you are saying.
- Reassure the resident. Tell him or her that you will provide protection from harm.
- Distract the resident with some item or activity.
- Use touch to calm and reassure the resident.

Comfort, rest, and sleep

- Provide good skin care. Make sure the resident's skin is free of urine and feces.
- Promote urinary and bowel elimination.

Comfort, rest, and sleep—cont'd

- Promote exercise and activity during the day. This helps reduce wandering and sundowning behaviors. The resident may also sleep better.
- Check with the nurse about reducing the resident's intake of coffee, tea, and cola drinks. These contain caffeine, which can increase the resident's restlessness, confusion, and agitation.
- Provide a quiet, restful environment. Soft music is better in the evening than loud television programs.
- Promote personal hygiene. Do not force the resident into a shower or tub. Residents with Alzheimer's disease are often afraid of bathing. Try bathing when the resident is calm.
- Provide oral hygiene.
- Have hygiene equipment ready ahead of time for any procedure. This reduces the amount of time the resident has to be involved in care measures.

care for the resident. Anger and resentment may result. The family may then feel guilty because of their anger and resentment. They know that the resident did not choose to develop the disease. The family also knows that the resident does not choose to have the signs, symptoms, and behaviors of the disease. They may be frustrated and angry that the loved one is no longer able to show love or affection. Sometimes the resident's behavior is embarrassing.

The family has to learn some of the same care and procedures that nurse aides learn. They need to learn how to bathe, feed, dress, and give oral hygiene to the resident. They also need to learn how to provide a safe environment. The nurse and support group will help them learn to give necessary care. Many of the measures described in the box may be part of the resident's care plan.

SUMMARY

Dementia affects a resident's ability to think, reason, and understand. Memory, judgment, and behavior are also affected. Therefore, dementia affects the ability to meet basic needs. Physical, safety, love and belonging, esteem, and self-actualization needs are all affected.

Residents with dementia do not choose to be forgetful, to wander, or to have poor manners. The disease is responsible for their behaviors. As frustrating as their behaviors may be, you must remember that they have no control over their actions.

The resident and family need much encouragement and emotional support. Required care can be physically, emotionally, and financially draining. There are no cures. However, a kind, caring nurse aide can be comforting.

CHAPTER 18

Basic Restorative Services

Objectives

Define activities of daily living (ADL)

Discuss nursing measures that promote residents to do their own activities of daily living

Explain why recreational activities are important for the elderly

Help a resident walk

Explain how to help a falling resident

Describe four walking aids

Describe range-of-motion (ROM) exercises

Describe bed rest

Identify the complications of bed rest

Describe the eight basic bed positions

Explain how to prevent muscle atrophy and contractures

Describe the devices used to support and maintain the body in alignment

Identify the uses of a trapeze

Describe a bladder retraining program

Describe a bowel retraining program

Being active is important for physical and psychological well-being. Disease, injury, and surgery can result in loss of bodily function or loss of a body part. Often there is loss of more than one function, which leads to some degree of activity limitation. The limitation effects everyday activities such as eating, bathing, dressing, grooming, and toileting. In addition to disabilities, even minimal inactivity can affect the normal functioning of every body system.

Health care is increasingly concerned with preventing and reducing the degree of disability and the effects of inactivity.

Nursing personnel are responsible for promoting exercise and activity in residents to the maximum degree possible. This process of restoring the disabled is called rehabilitation or restorative nursing. The nurse will instruct you about the resident's activity level and what exercises to perform.

ACTIVITIES OF DAILY LIVING

A major goal of rehabilitation is for the individual to be able to perform self-care activities. *Activities of daily living (ADL)* is the phrase used to refer to self-care activities. Activities of daily living are performed daily to remain independent and to function in society. These activities include bathing, oral hygiene, eating, bowel and bladder elimination, and moving about. A resident's ability to perform activities of daily living and the need for self-help devices are evaluated.

The hands, wrists, and arms may be affected by disease or injury. Self-help devices may be needed for various activities. Equipment can be changed or developed to meet the individual's needs in most instances. Special eating utensils may be needed. Glass holders, plate guards, and silverware with curved handles or cuffs are available. A special splint may be needed to which devices can be attached (Fig. 18-1). Electric toothbrushes are helpful if the person is unable to perform the back-and-forth motions necessary for brushing teeth. Longer handles can be attached to combs, brushes, and sponges. Self-help devices are also available for preparing meals, using kitchen appliances, dressing, writing, dialing telephones, and for many other activities.

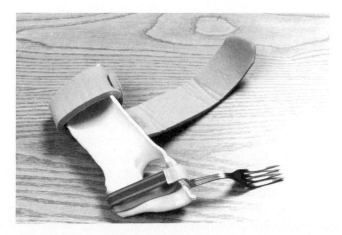

Fig. 18-1 Self help devices. *(From Sorrentino SA:* Mosby's textbook for nursing assistants, *ed 3, St Louis, 1992, Mosby–Year Book.)*

RECREATIONAL ACTIVITIES

Recreational activities are important for the persons in nursing facilities. The activities are important physically and psychologically. Joints and muscles are exercised and circulation is stimulated. Recreational activities also provide social opportunities and are mentally stimulating.

Bingo, movies, dances, exercise groups, shopping trips, museum trips, concerts, and guest speakers are often arranged by nursing facilities. Some facilities have fashion shows, gourmet meal nights, family cook-outs, and gardening activities. Grade school and high school music groups often perform in nursing facilities.

Residents may need help getting to an activity. Some also need help in participating. You need to provide assistance as necessary.

AMBULATION

Most residents that are prescribed bed rest are able to increase activity. Activity is increased slowly and in steps. First the person dangles (sits on the side of the bed). The next step is to sit in a bedside chair. Next the person walks in parallel bars, about in the room, and then in the hallway. *Ambulation*, the act of walking, should not be a problem if complications have been prevented. Contractures and muscle atrophy are prevented by proper positioning and exercise.

Residents may be weak and unsteady from bed rest, surgery, injury or disability. Use a gait (transfer) belt to ambulate the resident. This is a safety device that is applied snuggly to the waist. The resident should wear shoes with non-skid soles. For additional support the resident can use the hand rails along the wall. After ambulating the resident, report how well the resident tolerated the activity and the distance walked (Fig. 18-2).

THE FALLING RESIDENT

Residents may begin to fall when standing or walking. They may be weak, lightheaded, or dizzy. Fainting may occur. Falling may be due to slipping or sliding on spills, waxed floors, throw rugs, or improper shoes. When a person is falling, there is a tendency to try to prevent the fall. However, trying to prevent a fall could cause greater harm. Twisting and straining to stop the fall could cause injuries to yourself and the resident. Head injuries and hip fractures are common from falls. Balance is lost as a resident is falling. If you try to prevent the fall, you could lose your balance. Thus both you and the resident could fall or cause the other person to fall.

If a resident begins to fall, ease him or her to the floor grasping the transfer belt and allowing the resident to slide down your leg. This lets you control the direction of the fall. You can also protect the resident's head (Fig. 18-3). Call a nurse to check the resident. Report the distance walked, any complaints prior to the fall, the resident's pulse before the walk, and the amount of assistance needed by the resident while walking.

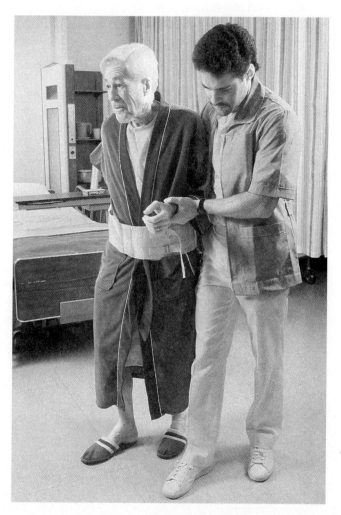

Fig. 18-2 Nurse aide walks at resident's side during ambulation. A transfer belt is used for the resident's safety. *(From Sorrentino SA:* Mosby's textbook for nursing assistants, *ed 3, St Louis, 1992, Mosby–Year Book.)*

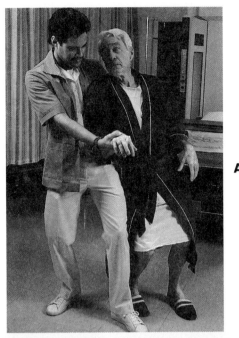

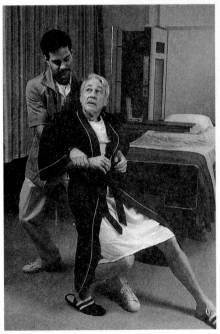

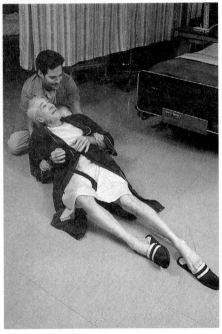

Fig. 18-3 A, Supporting the falling resident. **B,** The resident's buttocks are on the nurse aide's leg. **C,** The resident is eased to the floor on the nurse aide's leg. *(From Sorrentino SA: Mosby's textbook for nursing assistants, ed 3, St Louis, 1992, Mosby–Year Book.)*

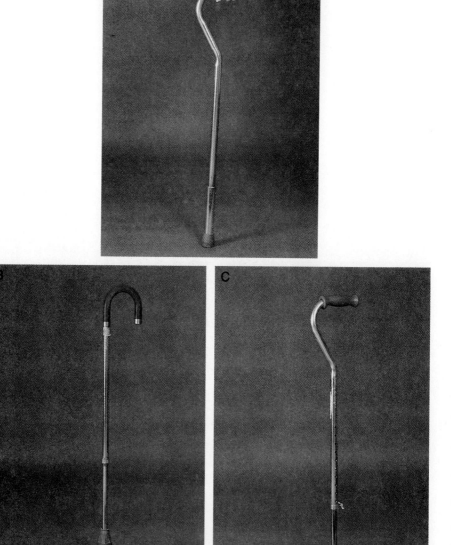

Fig. 18-4 A, Single tipped cane. **B,** Tri-pod cane. **C,** Four point (quad) cane. *(From Sorrentino SA:* Mosby's textbook for nursing assistants, *ed 3, St Louis, 1992, Mosby–Year Book.)*

WALKING AIDS (AMBULATION ASSISTIVE DEVICES)

Walking aids support the body. They are ordered by the doctor. The type ordered depends on the resident's physical condition, the amount of support needed, and the type of disability. The physical therapist and nurse teaches the resident to use the walking aid. It may be needed temporarily or permanently.

Canes

Canes are used when there is weakness on one side of the body. They provide balance and support. There are single-tipped canes and canes with three and four points (Fig. 18-4). A cane is held on the strong side of the body. (If the left leg is weak, the cane is held in the right hand). Three-point and four-point canes give more support than single-tipped canes. However, they are harder to move.

The tip of the cane should be about 6 to 10 inches (15 to 25 cm) to the side of the foot. The grip is level with the hip. When walking, the cane is moved first. It is moved forward about 12 inches. The weak leg (opposite the cane) is then moved forward even with the cane. Then the strong leg is brought forward and ahead of the cane and weak leg.

Walkers

A walker is a four-point walking aid (Fig. 18-5). It gives more support than a cane. Many people feel safer and more secure with a walker than with a cane. There

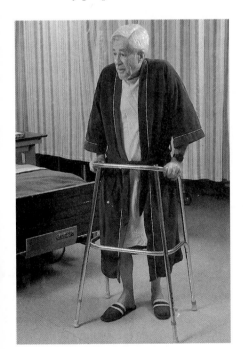

Fig. 18-5 A walker.
(*From Sorrentino SA:* Mosby's textbook for nursing assistants, *ed 3, St Louis, 1992, Mosby–Year Book.*)

are many kinds of walkers. The standard walker is picked up and moved about 6 inches in front of the resident. The resident then moves the right and then the left foot up to the walker. If the resident has a weak side, move the weak foot, then the strong foot up to the walker.

Baskets, pouches, and trays can be attached to walkers. The attachments allow people to carry needed items rather than rely on others to do so. This allows greater independence. The attachment also keeps hands free to grip the walker.

Braces

Braces and ankle foot orthoses (AFO) support weak body parts. They are also used to prevent or correct deformities or to prevent the movement of a joint. Metal, plastic, or leather are used for braces (Fig. 18-6). AFOs are made of plastic and velcro. These devices are applied to the foot and ankle. Bony points under braces and AFOs must be protected. Skin breakdown can occur.

Exercise

Exercise helps prevent contractures, muscle atrophy, and other complications of bed rest. Some exercise occurs with activities of daily living and when turning and moving in bed without assistance. However, additional exercises are needed for muscles and joints.

Trapeze. A trapeze or trapeze bar is a swinging bar suspended from an overbed frame (Fig. 18-7). The resident grasps the bar with both hands to lift the trunk off the bed. The trapeze is also used to move up and turn in bed. If allowed, it can be used for pulling exercises to strengthen the arm muscles.

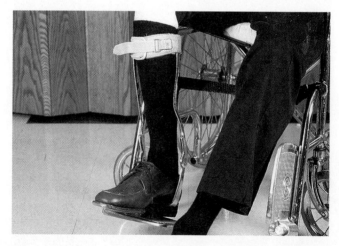

Fig. 18-6 Leg brace. (*From Sorrentino SA:* Mosby's textbook for nursing assistants, *ed 3, St Louis, 1992, Mosby–Year Book.*)

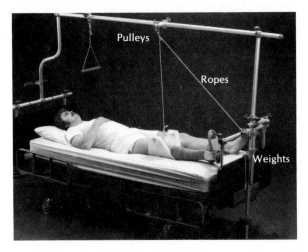

Fig. 18-7 Traction set-up with trapeze. (*From Perry AG, Potter PA:* Clinical nursing skills and techniques, *ed 2, St Louis, 1990, Mosby–Year Book.)*

Range-of-motion exercises. The movement of a joint to the extent possible without causing pain is the *range-of-motion (ROM)* of that joint. Range-of-motion exercises involve exercising the joints through their complete range-of-motion. The exercises are done at least twice a day (bid). Range-of-motion exercises may be active, passive, or active-assistive. *Passive* exercises involve having another person move the joints through their range-of-motion. *Active-assistive* range-of-motion is when the resident does the exercises with assistance from another person.

The following movements are involved in range-of-motion exercises.

Abduction—moving a body part away from the body
Adduction—moving a body part toward the body
Extension—straightening a body part
Flexion—bending a body part
Hyperextension—the excessive straightening of a body part
Dorsiflexion—bending backward
Rotation—turning the joint
Internal rotation—turning the joint inward
External rotation—turning the joint outward
Pronation—turning downward
Supination—turning upward
Radial-ulnarflexion—turning hand toward thumb; turning hand toward little
    finger
Thumb opposition—touch each finger tip with thumb

Range-of-motion exercises are done during activities of daily living. Residents on bed rest have few opportunities to be active. Therefore, range-of-motion exercises may be ordered. The nurse tells you which joints to exercise and if the exercises are to be active, passive, or active-assistive.

General rules. Range-of-motion exercises can cause injury if not performed properly. The following rules are practiced when performing or assisting with range-of-motion exercises.

1. Provide for the resident's safety and privacy.
2. Position the resident in the supine (backlying) position.
3. Exercise only the joints that the nurse tells you to exercise.
4. Expose only the body part being exercised.
5. Use good body mechanics.
6. Support the extremity being exercised at the joints.
7. Move the joint slowly, smoothly, and gently; perform each motion three times.
8. Do not force a joint beyond its present range-of-motion or the point of pain.
9. Exercise the body from head to toe performing the following exercises:
   A. Neck—flexion, extension, rotation (Fig. 18-8).
   B. Shoulder—flexion, extension, abduction, adduction, internal and external rotation, horizontal abduction, adduction (Fig. 18-9).
   C. Forearm and elbow—flexion, extension, supination, pronation (Figs. 18-10 and 18-11).
   D. Wrist—flexion, extension, hyperextension, radial-ulnarflexion (Fig. 18-12).
   E. Fingers—flexion, extension, abduction, adduction (Fig. 18-13).
   F. Thumb—flexion, extension, abduction, adduction, opposition and rotation (Fig. 18-14).
   G. Hip—flexion, extension, abduction, adduction, internal and external rotation (Fig. 18-15).
   H. Knee—flexion, extension (Fig. 18-16).
   I. Ankle—dorsiflexion (bending foot back), plantarflexion (bending foot down) (Fig. 18-17).
   J. Foot—supination, pronation (Fig. 18-18).
   K. Toes—flexion, extension, abduction, adduction (Fig. 18-19).

Text continued on p. 265.

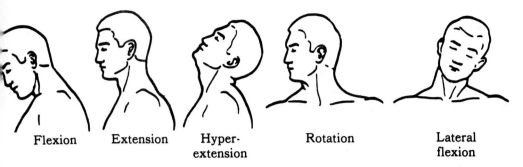

Flexion   Extension   Hyper-extension   Rotation   Lateral flexion

Fig. 18-8 Range-of-motion exercises for the neck. *(From Sorrentino SA:* Mosby's textbook for nursing assistants, *ed 3, St Louis, 1992, Mosby–Year Book.)*

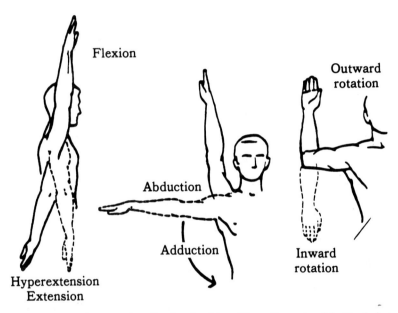

Flexion

Outward rotation

Abduction

Adduction

Inward rotation

Hyperextension
Extension

Fig. 18-9 Range-of-motion exercises for the shoulder. *(From Sorrentino SA:* Mosby's textbook for nursing assistants, *ed 3, St Louis, 1992, Mosby–Year Book.)*

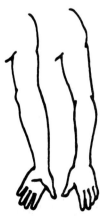

Supination   Pronation

Fig. 18-10 Range-of-motion exercises for the forearm. *(From Sorrentino SA:* Mosby's textbook for nursing assistants, *ed 3, St Louis, 1992, Mosby–Year Book.)*

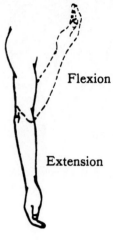

Fig. 18-11 Range-of-motion exercises for the elbow. *(From Sorrentino SA:* Mosby's textbook for nursing assistants, *ed 3, St Louis, 1992, Mosby–Year Book.)*

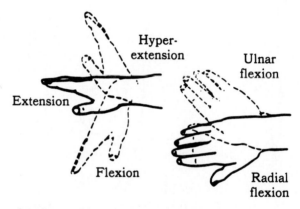

Fig. 18-12 Range-of-motion exercises for the wrist. *(From Sorrentino SA:* Mosby's textbook for nursing assistants, *ed 3, St Louis, 1992, Mosby–Year Book.)*

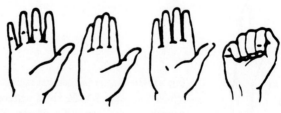

Abduction Adduction Extension Flexion

Fig. 18-13 Range-of-motion exercises for the fingers. *(From Sorrentino SA:* Mosby's textbook for nursing assistants, *ed 3, St Louis, 1992, Mosby–Year Book.)*

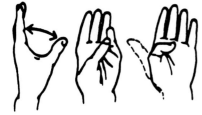

Abduction   Opposition   Extension
Adduction   to little   Flexion
         finger

Fig. 18-14 Range-of-motion exercises for the thumb. *(From Sorrentino SA:* Mosby's textbook for nursing assistants, *ed 3, St Louis, 1992, Mosby–Year Book.)*

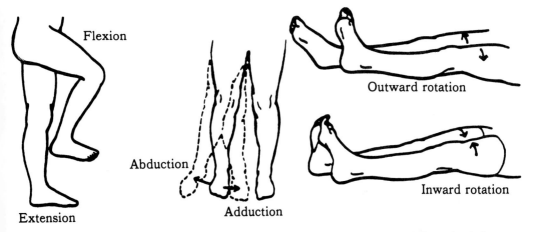

Flexion

Outward rotation

Abduction

Inward rotation

Extension

Adduction

Fig. 18-15 Range-of-motion exercises for the hip. *(From Sorrentino SA:* Mosby's textbook for nursing assistants, *ed 3, St Louis, 1992, Mosby–Year Book.)*

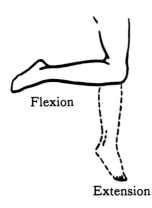

Flexion

Extension

Fig. 18-16 Range-of-motion exercises for the knee. *(From Sorrentino SA:* Mosby's textbook for nursing assistants, *ed 3, St Louis, 1992, Mosby– Year Book.)*

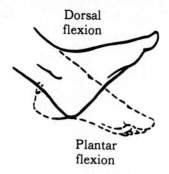

Fig. 18-17 Range-of-motion exercises for the ankle. *(From Sorrentino SA:* Mosby's textbook for nursing assistants, *ed 3, St Louis, 1992, Mosby–Year Book.)*

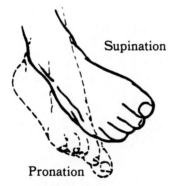

Fig. 18-18 Range-of-motion exercises for the foot. *(From Sorrentino SA:* Mosby's textbook for nursing assistants, *ed 3, St Louis, 1992, Mosby–Year Book.)*

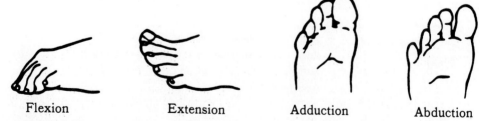

Fig. 18-19 Range-of-motion exercises for the toes. *(From Sorrentino SA:* Mosby's textbook for nursing assistants, *ed 3, St Louis, 1992, Mosby–Year Book.)*

BED REST

Bed rest has many meanings. The resident that has been prescribed bed rest may be allowed to participate in activities of daily living (ADL) such as bathing, oral hygiene, hair care, and feeding. If "strict" or "absolute" bed rest is ordered, everything is done for the resident. The resident is not allowed to perform any activities of daily living.

Bed rest may be ordered by the doctor because of a resident's health problem. You must know the activities that are allowed for each resident on bed rest. The nurse will provide this information.

The complications of bed rest and immobility

Bed rest has many useful purposes. The person is allowed to rest and does not have to move about as usual. Pain is reduced and healing promoted. However, bed rest and the lack of exercise and activity can cause serious complications. Decubitus ulcers, constipation, and fecal impaction can result. Blood clots, urinary tract infections, and pneumonia (infection of the lung) can also occur. Contractures and muscle atrophy are also complications of bed rest and immobility.

A *contracture* is the abnormal shortening of a muscle. The contracted muscle is fixed into position (Fig. 18-20), is permanently deformed, and cannot be stretched. The resident is permanently deformed and disabled. Contractures must be prevented. *Atrophy* is the decrease in size or the wasting away of tissue. Muscle atrophy is a decrease in size or a wasting away of the muscle. These complications must be prevented so normal body movement can occur.

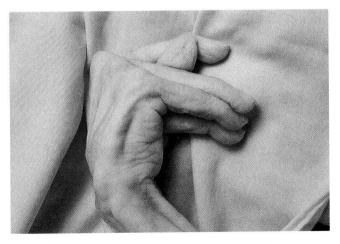

Fig. 18-20 A contracture. (*From Sorrentino SA:* Mosby's textbook for nursing assistants, *ed 3, St Louis, 1992, Mosby–Year Book.*)

Preventing the complications of bed rest

The complications of bed rest can be prevented by good nursing care. You have an important role in preventing contractures and muscle atrophy. Positioning in good body alignment is essential. Performing range-of-motion exercises is another important preventive measure.

Positioning in a chair

Residents who sit in chairs must be able to hold their upper bodies and heads erect. Poor alignment results if a resident is unable to stay in an erect position. The resident's back and buttocks should be up against the back of the chair. Feet should be flat on the floor or on the footrests of a wheelchair. The back of the knees and calves should be slightly away from the edge of the seat. With the nurse's permission, you can put a small pillow between the resident's lower back and the chair. This gives support to the lower back. Paralyzed arms are positioned on pillows. Wrists are positioned so that they are at a slight upward angle.

Residents may require postural supports if they are unable to keep their upper bodies erect. Postural supports help keep a resident in good body alignment. Besides positioning the resident in good body alignment, supportive devices may be necessary. They support and maintain a resident in a particular position.

Bed positions and positioning aids

There are eight basic bed positions—Fowler's, semi-Fowler's, Trendelenburg's, reverse Trendelenburg's, supine, prone, lateral, and Sim's.

Fowler's position is a semisitting position. The head of the bed is elevated 45 to 60 degrees (Fig. 18-21). Residents with respiratory and cardiac disorders are usually able to breathe easier in this position.

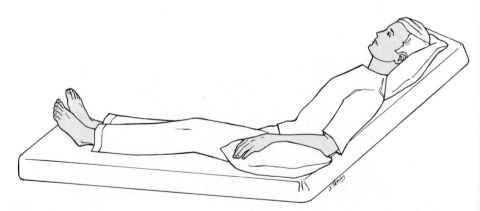

Fig. 18-21 Resident in a Fowler's position with pillows to maintain body alignment. (*From Sorrentino SA:* Mosby's textbook for nursing assistants, *ed 3, St Louis, 1992, Mosby–Year Book.*)

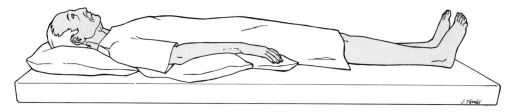

Fig. 18-22 Resident in a supine position. *(From Sorrentino SA:* Mosby's textbook for nursing assistants, *ed 3, St Louis, 1992, Mosby–Year Book.)*

In the *semi-Fowler's position* the head of the bed is raised 45 degrees and the knee portion is raised 15 degrees. This position is comfortable and prevents residents from sliding down in bed. However, raising the knee portion can interfere with circulation. Consult with the nurse before positioning a resident in the semi-Fowler's position.

Trendelenburg's position involves lowering the head of the bed and raising the foot of the bed. This position is used only when ordered by a doctor or nurse. Blocks are placed under the lower legs of the bed. Some beds are made so that the entire bedframe can be tilted into Trendelenburg's position.

Reverse Trendelenburg's position is the opposite of Trendelenburg's position. The head of the bed is elevated and the foot of the bed lowered. Blocks are put under the legs at the head of the bed or the bedframe is tilted. This position requires a doctor's order.

Supine position is the backlying position. Dorsal recumbent is another term used to mean the supine position. Good body alignment in this position involves having the bed flat, supporting the residents head and shoulders on a pillow, and placing the arms and hands at the resident's side. The resident's arms may be supported with regular-size pillows. The hands may be supported on small pillows with the palms down as in Fig. 18-22.

Residents in the *prone position* lie on their abdomens with their heads turned to one side. You can position the resident in good body alignment by placing a small pillow under the resident's head, one under the abdomen, and one under the lower legs (Fig. 18-23). The arms are flexed at the elbows with the hands near the head. You can also position residents so that their feet hang over the end of the mattress. If the feet hang over the mattress, a pillow is not needed under the lower legs.

A resident in the *lateral* or side-lying *position* lies on one side or the other (Fig. 18-24). Good body alignment for this position includes placing a pillow under the resident's head and shoulders and supporting the upper leg and thigh with pillows. A small pillow is placed under the upper hand and arm and a pillow is positioned against the resident's back.

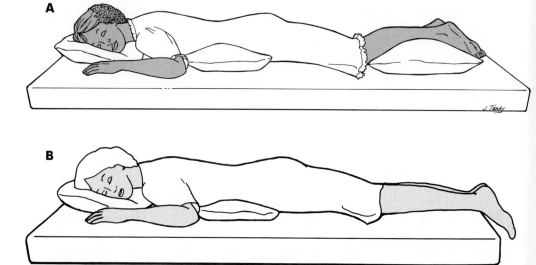

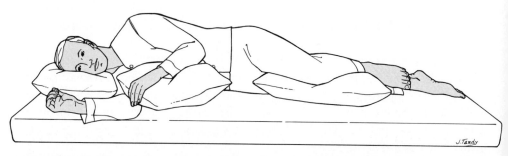

Fig. 18-23 A, Resident in a prone position. **B,** Resident in a prone position with feet hanging over the edge of the mattress. (*From Sorrentino SA:* Mosby's textbook for nursing assistants, *ed 3, St Louis, 1992, Mosby–Year Book.*)

Fig. 18-24 Resident in lateral position. (*From Sorrentino SA:* Mosby's textbook for nursing assistants, *ed 3, St Louis, 1992, Mosby–Year Book.*)

The *Sim's position* is a side-lying position. The upper leg is sharply flexed so that it is not on the lower leg, and the lower arm is behind the resident (Fig. 18-25). Good body alignment in this position involves placing a pillow under the head and shoulder, supporting the upper leg with a pillow, and placing a pillow under the upper arm and hand. In addition to the different bed positions, there are positioning aids help prevent the complications of bed rest.

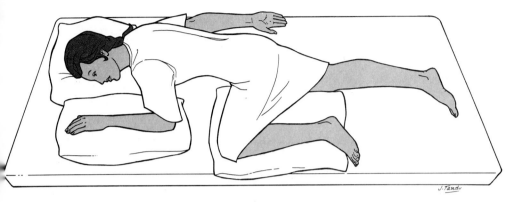

Fig. 18-25 Resident in Sim's position supported with pillows. *(From Sorrentino SA:* Mosby's textbook for nursing assistants, *ed 3, St Louis, 1992, Mosby–Year Book.)*

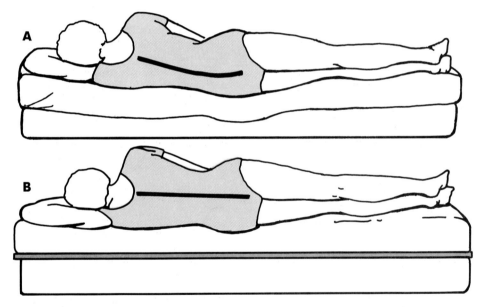

Fig. 18-26 A, Mattress sagging without bed boards. **B,** Bed boards placed under mattress. *(From Sorrentino SA:* Mosby's textbook for nursing assistants, *ed 3, St Louis, 1992, Mosby–Year Book.)*

Bed boards are placed under the mattress. They keep the resident in better alignment by preventing the mattress from sagging (Fig. 18-26). Bed boards are usually made of plywood and are covered with canvas or other material. They are made in two sections. One is for the head of the bed and the other for the foot. The two sections allow the head of the bed to be raised.

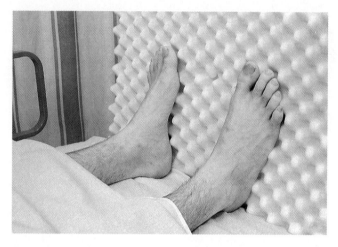

Fig. 18-27 Footboard. *(From Sorrentino SA:* Mosby's textbook for nursing assistants, *ed 3, St Louis, 1992, Mosby–Year Book.)*

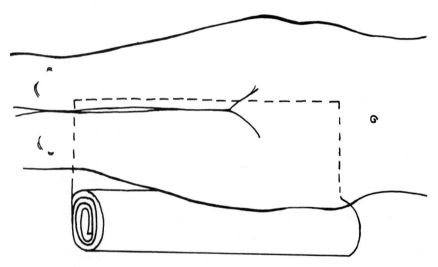

Fig. 18-28 Trochanter roll made from a bath blanket. *(From Sorrentino SA:* Mosby's textbook for nursing assistants, *ed 3, St Louis, 1992, Mosby–Year Book.)*

A *footboard* (Fig. 18-27) is placed at the foot of the mattress to prevent *plantar flexion (footdrop)*. In plantar flexion the foot *(plantar)* is bent *(flexion)*. The footboard is positioned so that the soles of the feet are flush against the footboard. The feet are in good body alignment as in the standing position. The footboard can be used as in the standing position. The footboard can be used as a bed cradle to keep top linens off of the feet.

Trochanter rolls (Fig. 18-28) prevent the hips and legs from turning outward (external rotation). Bath blankets are used for trochanter rolls. The blanket is folded to the desired length and rolled up. The loose end is placed under the resident from the hip to the knee. Then the roll is tucked along the side of the body. Pillows or sandbags can also be used to keep the hips and knees in alignment.

REHABILITATION
Bladder retraining

Bladder retraining programs may be developed for residents with urinary incontinence. Voluntary control of urination is the goal. With the doctor's approval, the nurse develops a plan to bladder train an individual. The bladder retraining program is part of the nursing care plan. You will assist in the program as directed by the nurse.

The basic method for bladder retraining is to have the resident use the toilet, commode, bedpan, or urinal at scheduled intervals. The resident is given 15 or 20 minutes to start voiding. The rules for helping to maintain normal urination are followed during bladder training. The normal position for urination should be assumed if possible. Privacy is important.

Bowel retraining

Bowel retraining involves two aspects. One is gaining control of bowel movements. The other is developing a regular pattern of elimination. Fecal impaction, constipation, and anal incontinence are prevented.

The urge to defecate is usually felt after a meal, particularly breakfast. Therefore, the use of the toilet, commode, or bedpan is encouraged at this time. Other factors that influence elimination are included in the nursing care plan and bowel training program. These include diet, high-fiber fluids, activity, and privacy. The nurse will give you instructions about an individual's bowel training program.

The physician may order a *suppository* to stimulate defecation. This is a cone-shaped, solid medication that is inserted into a body opening. It melts at body temperature. The rectal suppository is inserted into the rectum by the nurse. It is inserted about 30 minutes before the time selected for the bowel movement. Enemas may also be ordered.

Goals

The goals of the bowel and bladder retraining are:

1. Establish a regular elimination pattern.
2. Decrease or eliminate incontinent episodes.
3. Increase the resident's self-esteem.
4. Reduce the chances for skin breakdown.

Prosthetic devices

A prosthesis is an artificial replacement for a missing body part (for example, an eye or artificial limb). An individual usually can be fitted with an artificial arm or leg and taught how to use the prosthesis. Artificial eyes are available. Breast prostheses are available for women who have had a mastectomy (breast removal).

Psychological and social considerations

Self-esteem and relationships with others are often affected by a disability. Changes in body appearance and function may cause the resident to feel incomplete, unattractive, unclean, or undesirable to others. During the early stages of rehabilitation it is common for the individual to refuse to acknowledge the disability. The individual may become depressed, angry, and hostile.

A successful rehabilitation program depends on the resident's attitude, acceptance of limitations, and motivation. The individual needs to focus on remaining abilities. Feelings of discouragement and frustration are common. Progress may be slow or efforts unsuccessful. Each new task that must be learned is a reminder of the disability. Old fears and emotions may again be experienced. The individual needs help in accepting the disability and resulting limitations. Support, reassurance, encouragement, and sensitivity from members of the health team are necessary.

Economic considerations

The individual may be unable to return to former activities. The person is evaluated to determine work abilities, past work experiences, interests, and talents. The goal is for the individual to become as independent as possible.

SUMMARY

Exercise and activity are necessary for physical and psychological well-being. Complications from a lack of activity or exercise can occur when a person is confined to bed. You will position and exercise residents. Exercises prevent the complications of bed rest, especially muscle atrophy and contractures. Muscle atrophy can make ambulation difficult. A contracture results in loss of function and movement of the body part. A leg contracture may make normal ambulation impossible. Supportive devices and range-of-motion exercises also help prevent muscle atrophy and contractures.

The nurse aide should encourage the resident to do as much self-care activities as possible, such as bathing, grooming, dressing, and toileting. You should also report early signs and symptoms of complications of bed rest. A weak resident may need assistance in walking. Some people need walking aids on a permanent or temporary basis. Doctors may prescribe crutches, canes, walkers, or braces.

CHAPTER 19

Residents' Rights

Objectives

Describe residents' rights and how to promote a resident's quality of life.

Explain what is meant by elderly abuse and the signs of elderly abuse.

Explain what to do if you suspect elderly abuse.

RESIDENT RIGHTS

Residents of nursing facilities have certain rights under federal and state laws. Residents have rights as citizens of the United States. They also have rights relating to their everyday lives and care in a nursing facility. Nursing facilities must protect and promote resident rights. Residents must be able to exercise their rights without facility interference. Some residents are incompetent (not able) and cannot exercise their rights. Legal guardians exercise rights for them.

Nursing facilities must inform residents of their rights. They must be informed orally and in writing. Such information is given before or upon admission to the facility. It must be given in the language used and understood by the resident.

Privacy and confidentiality

The right to privacy and confidentiality in relation to resident information and records means that the resident should expect that information will be shared with health-care workers in a careful and wise manner. The information found in a resident's record should not go outside the facility. OBRA provides for confidentiality and privacy.

Information about the resident's care, treatment, and condition must be kept confidential. Medical and financial records are also confidential. The resident must give consent for them to be released to other facilities or individuals. However, consent is not needed for the release of medical records when the resident is being transferred to another facility. Records can also be released without the resident's consent when they are required by law or for insurance purposes.

Residents have the right to personal privacy. The resident's body must not be exposed unnecessarily. Only those workers directly involved in care, treatments, or examinations should be present. The resident must give consent for others to be present. A resident also has the right to use the bathroom in private. Privacy should also be maintained for personal care activities.

Residents also have the right to visit with others in privacy. They have the right to visit in an area where they cannot be seen or heard by others. The facility must try to provide private space for this when it is requested. Offices, chapels, dining rooms, meeting rooms, and conference rooms can be used if available.

The right to visit in privacy also involves telephone conversations. Residents also have the right to send and receive mail without interference by others. Letters sent and received by the resident must not be opened by others without the resident's permission.

Personal choice

OBRA requires that residents be free to choose their physicians. They also have the right to participate in planning their care and treatment. This means that residents have the right to choose activities, schedules, and care based on their personal preferences. For example, residents have the right to choose when to get up and go to bed, what to wear, how to spend their time, and what to eat. They can also choose companions and visitors inside and outside of the nursing facility.

Personal choice is important for quality of life, dignity, and self-respect. You will be reminded to allow the resident's preferences whenever it is safely possible.

Disputes and grievances

Residents have the right to voice concerns, questions, and complaints about treatment or care. The dispute or grievance may involve another resident, or it may be about treatment or care that was not given. The facility must promptly try to correct the situation. The resident must not be punished in any way for voicing the dispute or grievance.

Participation in resident and family groups

Residents have the right to participate in resident and family groups. This means that residents have the right to form groups. A resident's family has the right to meet with the families of other residents. These groups can discuss concerns and offer suggestions to improve quality of life in the facility. They can also plan activities for residents and families or the groups can serve to provide support and reassurance for group members. Residents also have the right to participate in social, religious, and community activities. Activities are provided regularly for residents in nursing facilities. They also have the right to assistance in getting to and from activities of their choice.

Care and security of personal possessions

Residents have the right to keep and use personal possessions. Available space and the health and safety of other residents can affect the type and amount of personal possessions allowed. A resident's property must be treated with care and respect. Though the items may not have value to you, they are important to the resident. They also relate to personal choice, dignity, and quality of life.

The facility must take reasonable measures to protect the individual's property. Items should be labelled with the resident's name. The facility must investigate reports of lost, stolen, or damaged items. Police assistance is sometimes necessary. The resident and family will probably be advised not to keep jewelry and other expensive items in the facility.

You must protect yourself and the facility from being accused of stealing a resident's property. Do not go through a resident's closet, drawers, purse, or other space without the resident's knowledge and consent. Have another worker with you and the resident or legal guardian present if it is necessary to inspect closets and drawers. The worker serves as a witness to your activities.

Freedom from abuse, mistreatment, and neglect

OBRA states that residents have the right to be free from verbal, sexual, physical, or mental abuse. Elderly abuse is discussed later in this chapter.

Residents also have the right to be free from involuntary seclusion. Involuntary seclusion is separating the resident from others against his or her will. It can also mean keeping the resident away from his or her room without consent, or being confined to a certain area. If the person is competent, involuntary seclusion occurs against the legal guardian's consent.

No one can abuse, neglect, or mistreat the resident. This includes facility staff, volunteers, staff from other agencies or groups, other residents, family, visitors, and legal guardians. Nursing facilities must have policies and procedures for investigating suspected or reported cases of resident abuse. Also, nursing facilities cannot employ individuals who have been convicted for abusing, neglecting, or mistreating other individuals.

Freedom from restraints

Residents have the right not to have body movements restricted. Body movements can be restricted by the application of restraints or the administration of certain drugs. Some drugs can restrain the person because they affect mood, behavior, and mental function. Sometimes residents need to be restrained to protect them from harming themselves or others. These restraints may be physical or chemical. Physical restraints are made of cloth or leather. Chemical restraints are sedatives used to control aggressive behavior. A physician's order is necessary for restraints to be used. Restraints cannot be used for the convenience of the staff. Restraints are protective devices used to prevent the resident from injuring self or others. Safety principles that must be followed when using restraints include:

1. Restraints are used to protect residents.
2. Restraints require a physician's order.
3. Restraints are not to be used unnecessarily.
4. Basic needs must be met by the nurse aides.
5. Apply padding under a restraint as needed to prevent skin irritation.
6. Apply the restraint snugly, but allow sufficient room for movement.
7. Check restraints to insure adequate circulation.
8. Tie restraints with a square knot for easy release.
9. Remove restraints and reposition the resident at least every 2 hours.
10. Report and record the type of restraint, when it was applied, color and condition of resident's skin, and the presence of a pulse.

Quality of life

OBRA requires that nursing facilities care for residents in a manner that promotes dignity and self-esteem, as well as physical, psychological, and emotional well-being. Protecting resident rights is one way to promote quality of life. Personal choice, privacy, participation in group activities, personal property, and freedom of restraint are some ways which show respect for the resident.

The resident should also be spoken to in a polite and courteous manner. Giving good, honest, and thoughtful care will enhance the resident's quality of life.

Activities

Activities are also important for a resident's quality of life. OBRA requires that nursing facilities provide activity programs which meet the interests and physical, mental, and psychosocial needs of each resident. Such activities must allow personal choice and promote physical, intellectual, social, and emotional well-being. Many facilities also provide religious services for spiritual health. You will be responsible for assisting residents to and from activity programs. You may also be assigned to help residents with activities.

Environment

The environment of the facility must also promote quality of life. The environment must be clean and safe and be as homelike as possible. Allowing the resident to have personal possessions enhances quality of life by allowing personal choice and promoting a homelike environment.

ABUSE OF THE ELDERLY

Elderly abuse has become more evident in today's society. The abuser is usually a family member or a person caring for the elderly individual. The person may be intentionally harmed. There are different forms of abuse, which are described in the list below.

1. *Physical abuse* involves hitting, slapping, kicking, pinching, and beating. Physical injury and pain may result. This can also include depriving the person of needed medical services or treatment.
2. *Verbal abuse* can be described as the use of oral or written words or statements that speak ill of, sneer at, criticize, or condemn the resident. OBRA guidelines also include unkind gestures under verbal abuse.
3. *Involuntary seclusion* is confining the person to a specific area. Elderly people have been locked in closets, basements, attics, and other spaces.
4. *Financial abuse* is when the elderly person's money is used by another person.
5. *Mental abuse* relates to humiliation and threats of being punished or deprived of such things as food, clothing, care, a home, or a place to sleep.
6. *Sexual abuse* is when a person is harassed about sex or is attacked sexually. The person may be forced to perform sexual acts out of fear of punishment or physical harm.

Abused elderly may be seen in their homes, hospitals, or nursing facilities. Often the abuse is unrecognized. There are many signs of elderly abuse. The abused person may show only some of the signs.

1. Living conditions are unsafe, unclean, or inadequate.
2. Personal hygiene is lacking. The individual is unclean and clothes are dirty.
3. Weight loss has occured. There are signs of poor nutrition and inadequate fluid intake.
4. There are frequent injuries. The circumstances behind the injuries are strange or seem impossible.
5. Old and new bruises are seen.
6. The person seems very quiet or withdrawn.
7. The person seems fearful, anxious, or agitated.
8. The individual does not seem to want to talk or answer questions.
9. The person is restrained or locked in a certain area for long periods of time. Toilet facilities, food, water, and other necessary items cannot be reached.
10. Private conversations are not allowed. The caregiver is present during all conversations.
11. The person seems too anxious to please the caregiver.
12. Medications are not taken properly. Medications are not purchased, or too much or too little medication is taken.
13. Visits to the emergency room may be frequent.
14. The person may go from one doctor to another, or the person does not have a doctor.

OBRA and state laws require the reporting of elderly abuse. If abuse is suspected, it must be reported. Where and how to report suspected abuse varies in each state. If you need to report suspected abuse, give as much information as possible. The reporting agency will take action based on the information given. They act immediately if there is a life-threatening situation. Sometimes the help of police or the courts is necessary.

Helping the abused elderly is not always easy or possible. The abuse may never be reported or recognized, or the investigating agency may be unable to gain access to the person. Sometimes the elderly are abused by their children. A victim may want to protect the child. Some victims are embarrassed or feel that the abuse is deserved. A victim may be afraid of what will happen. He or she may feel that the present situation is better than no care at all. Some people feel they will not be believed if they report the abuse themselves.

Elderly abuse is an unfortunate situation. You may suspect that a person is being abused. If so, discuss the situation and your observations with your supervisor. Give the nurse as much information as possible. The nurse will then contact the appropriate members of the health team. The agency which investigates elderly abuse in your community will also be contacted.

SUMMARY

OBRA protects individuals in nursing facilities. Some of the many OBRA requirements relate to resident rights and the quality of life.

Some elderly are abused. Their needs and problems present additional concerns. You must be alert to the possibility that a person is being abused. You can help the victim by discussing the situation with a nurse as soon as possible.

GLOSSARY _____

abduction Moving a body part away from the body

abuse Improper use of equipment, a substance, or a service, such as a drug or program, either intentionally or unintentionally

acetone Ketone bodies that appear in the urine because of the rapid breakdown of fat for energy

activities of daily living Those self-care activities a person needs to perform daily to remain independent and function in society

acute illness An illness that occurs suddenly and from which the patient is expected to recover

adduction Moving a body part toward the body

alimentary canal The long tube extending from the mouth to the anus; also called the gastrointestinal tract

AM care The routine care performed before breakfast; early morning care

amputation The removal of all or part of an extremity

anal incontinence The inability to control the passage of feces and gas through the anus

antiperspirant A skin care product that reduces the amount of perspiration

aphasia The loss of or inability (*a*) to speak (*phasia*)

apical-radial pulse Taking the apical pulse and the radial pulse at the same time; two workers are needed for the procedure

apnea The lack or absence of (*a*) breathing (*pnea*)

artery A blood vessel that carries blood away from the heart

arthritis Joint (*arthur*) inflammation (*itis*)

asepsis The absence of pathogens

aspiration The breathing of fluid or an object into the lungs

assault Intentionally attempting or threatening to touch the body of another person without the person's consent

atrophy A decrease in size or a wasting away of tissue

autoclave A pressurized steam sterilizer

autonomic nervous system A division of the peripheral nervous system; the system controls involuntary muscles and functions that occur without conscious effort

bacteria Microscopic one-celled plant life that multiplies rapidly; germs

base of support The area on which an object rests

bath blanket A thin, light-weight cotton blanket used to cover the patient during the bath; it absorbs water and provides warmth during the bath; it is used to cover the patient during many other procedures

battery The actual unauthorized touching of another person's body without the person's consent

bedsore A decubitus ulcer; a pressure sore

benign tumor   A tumor that grows slowly and within a localized area; benign tumors usually do not cause death

blood pressure   The amount of force exerted against the walls of an artery by the blood

body alignment   The way the body segments are aligned with one another; posture

body language   Facial expressions, gestures, posture, and other body movements that send messages to others

body mechanics   Using the body in an efficient and careful way

body temperature   The amount of heat in the body that is a balance between the amount of heat produced and the amount lost by the body

bradypnea   Slow *(brady)* breathing *(pnea);* the respiratory rate is less than 10 respirations per minute

braille   A method of writing for the blind; raised dots are arranged to represent each letter of the alphabet; the first ten letters also represent the numbers 0 through 9

calorie   The amount of energy produced from the burning of food for energy

capillary   The smallest blood vessel; food, oxygen, and other substances pass from the capillaries to the cells

cardiac arrest   The sudden stoppage of breathing and heart action

carrier   A human being or animal that is a reservoir for microorganisms but does not have the signs and symptoms of an infection

cartilage   The connective tissue at the end of long bones

caster   A small wheel made of rubber or plastic

catheter   A tube used to drain or inject fluid through a body opening

catheterization   The process of inserting a catheter

cell   The basic unit of body structure

cell membrane   The outer covering that encloses the cell and helps the cell hold its shape

central nervous system   One of two main divisions of the nervous system; made up of the brain and spinal cord

chart   Another term for the patient's record

Cheyne-Stokes   A pattern for breathing in which respirations gradually increase in rate and depth and then become shallow and slow; breathing may stop (apnea) for 10 to 20 seconds

chronic illness   An illness that is slow or gradual in onset and for which there is no known cure; it can be controlled, and complications can be prevented

chyme   Partially digested food and fluids that pass from the stomach into the small intestine

civil law   Laws concerned with the relationships among people; private law

clean technique   A term for medical asepsis

closed fracture   A fracture in which the bone is broken but the skin is intact; a simple fracture

colostomy   The surgical creation of an artificial opening between the colon and abdomen

coma   A state of being completely unaware of one's surroundings; the individual is unable to react or respond to people, places, or things

communicable disease   A disease caused by pathogens that are spread easily; a contagious disease

communication   The exchange of information; a message is sent, and it is received and interpreted by the intended person

complete bed bath   Washing the entire body of a resident who is in bed

compound fracture   An open fracture; the bone is broken and the bone has come through the skin

constipation   The passage of a hard, dry stool

constrict   To narrow

contagious disease   A communicable disease

contamination   The process by which an object or area becomes unclean

contracture   The abnormal shortening of a muscle

crime   An act that is a violation of a criminal law

criminal law   Laws concerned with offenses against the public and society in general; criminal law is also called public law

culture   The values, beliefs, habits, likes, dislikes, customs, and characteristics of a group that are passed from one generation to the next

dangling   Sitting on the side of the bed; sitting on the side of the bed and moving the legs back and forth and around in circles

decubitus ulcer   An areas where the skin and underlying tissues are eroded as a result of a lack of blood flow; a bedsore or pressure sore

defamation   Injuring the name and reputation of another person by making false statements to a third person

defecation   The process of excreting feces from the rectum through the anus; a bowel movement

dehydration   A decrease in the amount of water in body tissues

delusion   A false belief

dementia   The term used to describe mental disorders caused by changes in the brain

deodorant   A preparation that masks and controls body odors

dermis   The inner layer of the skin

development   Changes in a person's psychological and social functioning

developmental task   That which the individual must accomplish during a stage of development

diabetes mellitus   A chronic disease in which the pancreas fails to secrete enough insulin; the body is prevented from using sugar for energy

diarrhea   The frequent passage of liquid stools

diastole   The resting phase of heart action during which the heart fills with blood; the period of heart muscle relaxation

diastolic pressure   The pressure in the arteries when the heart is at rest

digestion   The process of physically and chemically breaking down food so that it can be absorbed for use by the cells of the body

dilate   To expand or open wider

disaster   A sudden, catastrophic event in which many people are injured or killed and property is destroyed

disinfection   The process by which pathogens are destroyed

dorsal recumbent position   The back-lying or supine position

dorsiflexion   Bending backward

drawsheet A sheet, smaller in size than a bottom or top sheet, that is placed over the middle of the bottom sheet; it helps keep the mattress and bottom linens clean and dry; it can also be used to turn and move residents in bed; it is sometimes called the "cotton drawsheet"

dysphagia Difficulty or discomfort *(dys)* in swallowing *(phagia)*

dyspnea Difficult, labored, or painful *(dys)* breathing *(pnea)*

dysuria Painful or difficult *(dys)* urination *(uria)*

early morning care AM care

edema The swelling of body tissues with water

enema The introduction of fluid into the rectum and lower colon

epidermis The outer layer of the skin

esteem The worth, value, or opinion one has of a person

ethics What is right and wrong conduct

exhalation The act of breathing out; expiration

extension Straightening of a body part

external rotation Turning the joint outward

fainting The sudden loss of consciousness caused by an inadequate blood supply to the brain

false imprisonment The unlawful restraint or restriction of another person's movement

fecal impaction The prolonged retention and accumulation of fecal material in the rectum

feces The semisolid mass of waste products in the colon

flatulence The excessive formation of gas in the stomach and intestines

flatus The gas or air in the stomach or intestines

flexion Bending a body part

Foley catheter A catheter that is left in the urinary bladder so that urine drains continuously into a collection bag; an indwelling or retention catheter

footdrop Plantar flexion

Fowler's position A semi-sitting position in which the head of the bed is elevated 45 to 60 degrees

fracture A broken bone

fracture pan A bedpan that has a thin rim and is more shallow at one end than normal bedpans

friction The rubbing of one surface against another

gait belt A transfer belt

gangrene A condition in which there is death of tissue; tissues become black, cold, and shriveled

gastrostomy Surgically created opening in the stomach that allows feeding

germs Bacteria

glucosuria Sugar *(glucos)* in the urine *(uria)*

graduate A calibrated container used to measure amounts of fluid

ground That which carries leaking electricity to the earth and away from the electrical appliance

growth The physical changes that can be measured and that occur in a steady, orderly manner

hallucination   Seeing, hearing, or feeling something that is not real

health team   A variety of health care workers who work together to provide health care for patients

hearing aid   An instrument that amplifies sound

hemiplegia   Paralysis on one side of the body

hemorrhage   The excessive loss of blood from a blood vessel

home health agency   An agency that provides nursing care and assistance to residents in their homes

horizontal recumbent position   The supine or back-lying examination position; the edges are together

hormone   A chemical substance secreted by glands into the bloodstream

hospice   A health care facility or program designed for individuals who are dying of terminal illness

hospital   A health care facility where ill and injured persons are given health care, including medical and nursing care

host   The environment in which the microorganism lives and grows; reservoir

hs care   Care given to the patient in the evening at bedtime

hyperextension   Excessive straightening of a body part

hypertension   Persistent blood pressure measurements above the normal systolic (150 mm Hg) or diastolic (90 mm Hg) pressures

hyperventilation   Respirations are rapid and deeper than normal

hypotension   A condition in which the systolic blood pressure is below 100 mm Hg and the diastolic pressure is below 60 mm Hg

hypoventilation   Respirations are slow, shallow, and sometimes irregular

ileostomy   The surgical creation of an artificial opening between the ileum (small intestine) and the abdomen

indwelling catheter   A retention, or Foley, catheter

infection   A disease state that results from the invasion and growth of microorganisms in the body

infection precautions   Practices that limit the spread of pathogens; barriers are set up that prevent the escape of the pathogen

inhalation   The act of breathing in; inspiration

integumentary system   The skin

internal rotation   Turning the joint inward

intravenous therapy   The fluid administered through a needle within (*intra*) a vein (*venous*); IV and IV infusion

invasion of privacy   A violation of a person's right not to have one's name, photograph, or private affairs exposed or made public without giving consent

joint   The point at which two or more bones meet

Kardex   A type of card file that summarizes the information contained in the resident's record; medications, treatments, diagnosis, routine care measures, and special equipment needed by the resident are included

ketone body   Acetone; it appears in the urine because of the rapid breakdown of fat for energy

knee-chest position The resident kneels and rests the body on the knees and chest; the head is turned to one side, the arms are above the head or flexed at the elbows, the back is straight, and the body is flexed about 90 degrees at the hips

lateral position The side-lying position

law A rule of conduct made by a government body

legal That which pertains to a law

liable Being responsible for one's own action

libel Defamation through written statements

licensed practical nurse (LPN) An individual who has completed a 1-year nursing program and has passed the licensing examination for practical nurses; the LPN assists the registered nurse in planning, giving, and evaluating nursing care; licensed vocational nurse (LVN) is the title used in some states

ligament A strong band of connective tissue that holds bones together

logrolling Turning the resident as a unit, in alignment, with one motion

long-term care facility A broad term used to describe a health care facility in which individuals live and are given nursing care; most residents are elderly and unable to care for themselves because of aging or illness

malignant tumor A tumor that grows rapidly and invades other tissues; malignant tumors will cause death if not treated

malpractice Negligence by a professional person

meatus The opening at the end of the urethra

medical asepsis The techniques and practices used to prevent the spread of pathogens from one person or place to another person or place; clean technique

menarche The time when menstruation first begins

meninges The connective tissue that covers and protects the brain and spinal cord; there are three layers: the outer layer called the dura mater, the middle layer called the arachnoid, and the inner layer called the pia mater

menopause The time when menstruation stops; it marks the end of the woman's reproductive years

menstruation The process in which the endometrium of the uterus breaks up and is discharged from the body through the vagina

mental health hospital A hospital for persons who are mentally ill

metabolism The burning of food for heat and energy for use by the cells

metastasis The spread of cancer to other parts of the body

microbe A microorganism

microorganism A small living plant or animal that cannot be seen without the aid of a microscope; a microbe

micturition The process of emptying the bladder; urination or voiding

mitered corner A way of tucking linens under the mattress to keep the linens straight and smooth

morning care Care that is given after breakfast; cleanliness and skin care measures are more thorough at this time

need That which is necessary or desirable for maintaining life and mental well-being

negligence   An unintentional wrong in which a person fails to act in a reasonable and prudent manner and thereby causes harm to another person or the person's property

nonpathogen   A microorganism that does not usually cause an infection

nonverbal communication   Communication that does not involve the use of words

normal flora   Microorganisms that usually live and grow in a certain location

nucleus   The control center of the cell that directs the cell's activities

nurse aide   An individual who gives simple, basic nursing care under the supervision of an RN or LPN; training may be received through a nursing assistant course, in-service program, or on-the-job training; other titles are nursing assistant, nursing attendant, and resident care assistant

nursing care plan   A written guide that gives direction about the care a resident should receive

nursing team   The individuals involved in providing nursing care; RNs, LPNs, and nursing assistants make up the nursing team

nutrient   A substance that is ingested, digested, absorbed, and used by the body

nutrition   The many processes involved in the ingestion, digestion, absorption, and use of foods and fluids by the body

objective data   Information observed about a patient that can be seen, heard, felt, or smelled by another person; signs

observation   Using the senses of sight, hearing, touch, and smell to collect information about the resident

open fracture   A fracture in which the bone is broken and the bone has come through the skin; a compound fracture

ophthalmoscope   A lighted instrument used to examine the internal structures of the eye

oral hygiene   The measures that are performed to keep the mouth and teeth clean; mouth care

orderly   A male nursing assistant

organ   Groups of tissues with the same function

ostomy   The surgical creation of an artificial opening

paraplegia   Paralysis from the waist down

partial bed bath   Bathing the resident's face, hands, axillae, genital area, back, and buttocks

pathogen   A microorganism that is harmful and is capable of causing an infection

pericare   Perineal care

perineal care   Cleansing the genital and anal areas of the body

peristalsis   Involuntary muscle contractions in the digestive system that move food through the alimentary canal; the alternating contraction and relaxation of the intestinal muscles

phantom limb pain   A sensation causing the resident to complain of pain in an amputated part; it may feel as if the part is still there

plantar flexion   The foot (*plantar*) is bent (*flexion*); footdrop

plasma   The fluid portion of the blood

plastic drawsheet   A drawsheet made of plastic, placed between the bottom sheet and the cotton drawsheet; it helps keep the mattress and bottom linens clean and dry; some are made of rubber and are called "rubber drawsheets"

postmortem   After *(post)* death *(mortem)*

posture   The way the body segments are aligned with one another; body alignment

pressure sore   A decubitus ulcer; a bedsore

pronation   Turning downward

prosthesis   An artificial placement for a missing body part

pulse   The beat of the heart felt at an artery as a wave of blood passes through the artery

pulse deficit   The difference between the apical and radial pulse rates

pulse rate   The number of hearbeats or pulses felt in 1 minute

pupil   The opening in the middle of the eye

quadriplegia   Paralysis from the neck down; paralysis of the arms, legs, and trunk

range of motion   The movement of a joint to the extent possible without causing pain

reality orientation   A form of rehabilitation aimed at promoting or maintaining awareness of person, time, and place

recording   Writing or charting resident care and observations

reflex   An involuntary movement

registered nurse (RN)   An individual who has studied nursing for 2, 3, or 4 years and has passed a licensing examination; the RN is responsible for assessing, planning, implementing, and evaluating nursing care

rehabilitation   The process of restoring the disabled individual to the highest level of physical, psychological, social, and economic functioning possible

reincarnation   The belief that the spirit or soul is reborn into another human body or into another form of life

religion   Spiritual beliefs, needs, and practices

reporting   A verbal account of patient care and observations

reservoir   The environment in which microorganisms live and grow; the host

resident record   A written account of the resident's illness and response to the treatment and care given by members of the health team; it is commonly referred to as a chart

resident pack   Personal care equipment provided by the health care facility; the pack generally includes a wash basin, emesis or kidney basin, bedpan, urinal, water pitcher and glass, soap, and a soap dish

resident unit   The furniture and equipment provided for the individual by the health care facility

respiration   The process of supplying the cells with oxygen and removing carbon dioxide from them; the act of breathing air into (inhalation) and out of (exhalation) the lungs

responsibility   A duty; an obligation to perform some act or function; being able to answer for one's actions

restraint   A device used in aiding the immobilization of residents

retention catheter   A Foley or indwelling catheter

reverse Trendelenburg's position   The head of the bed is elevated and the foot of the bed is lowered

rigor mortis   The stiffness or rigidity *(rigor)* of skeletal muscles that occurs after death *(mortis)*

self-actualization   Experiencing one's potential

semi-Fowler's position   The head of the bed is elevated 45 degrees and the knee portion is elevated 15 degrees; or the head of the bed is elevated 30 degrees and the knee portion is not elevated

sex   The physical activities involving the organs of reproduction; the activities are done for pleasure or to produce children

sexuality   That which relates to one's sex; those physical, psychological, social, culture, and spiritual factors that affect a person's feelings and attitudes about his or her sex

shock   A condition that results when there is an inadequate blood supply to the organs and tissues of the body

side-lying position   The lateral position

signs   Objective data

simple fracture   A closed fracture; the bone is broken but the skin is intact

Sims' position   A side-lying position in which the upper leg is sharply flexed so that it is not resting on the lower leg, and the lower arm is behind the patient

slander   Defamation through oral statements

sphygmomanometer   The instrument used to measure blood pressure that consists of a cuff (which is applied to the upper arm) and a measuring device

spore   A bacterium protected by a hard shell that forms around the microorganism

sputum   Mucus secreted by the lungs, bronchi, and trachea during respiratory illnesses or disorders

sterile   The absence of all microorganisms, both pathogenic and nonpathogenic

sterilization   The process by which all microorganisms are destroyed

stethoscope   An instrument used to listen to the sounds produced by the heart, lungs, and other body organs

stoma   An opening; see *colostomy* and *ileostomy*

stomatitis   Inflammation (*itis*) of the mouth (*stomat*)

stool   Feces that have been excreted

stroke   A cerebrovascular accident; blood supply to a part of the brain is suddenly interrupted

subjective data   Information reported by the resident that the health care worker cannot observe by using the senses; symptoms are subjective data

suction   The process of withdrawing or sucking up fluids

suffocation   The termination of breathing that results from lack of oxygen

sundowning   Condition in which signs, symptoms, and behaviors that are characteristic of Alzheimer's disease increase during hours of darkness

supination   Turning upward

supine position   The back-lying or dorsal recumbent position

suppository   A cone-shaped solid medication that is inserted into a body opening; the medication melts at body temperature

symptoms   Subjective data

system   Organs that work together to perform special functions

systole   The phase of heart action during which the heart contracts; the period of heart muscle contraction

systolic pressure The amount of force it takes to pump blood out of the heart into the arterial circulation

tachypnea Rapid *(tachy)* breathing *(pnea);* the respiratory rate is greater than 24 respirations per minute

terminal illness An illness or injury for which there is no reasonable expectation of recovery

tissue Groups of cells with the same function

toothette A piece of spongy foam attached to a stick that is used for giving oral hygiene

transfer belt A belt used to hold onto a resident during a transfer or when walking with the resident; a gait belt

Trendelenburg's position The head of the bed is lowered and the foot of the bed is raised

tumor A new growth of cells; tumors can be benign or malignant

turning sheet A flat sheet folded in half, or a drawsheet, that is used to lift, turn, or move a patient in bed; a lift or pull sheet

urethra The structure through which urine passes from the bladder and is eliminated from the body

urinary incontinence The inability to control the passage of urine from the bladder

urination The process of emptying the bladder; micturition or voiding

vein A blood vessel that carries blood back to the heart

verbal communication Communication that uses the written or spoken word

virus An extremely small microscopic organism that grows in living cells

vital signs Temperature, pulse, respirations, and blood pressure

voiding Urination or micturition

vomiting The act of expelling stomach contents through the mouth

will A legal declaration of how an individual wishes to have property distributed after death

INDEX ————————————

A

Abduction, 259
ABK, 112
Above-the-knee amputation, 112
Abuse
　of elderly, 51-53, 276-278
　freedom from, resident's right to, 51, 275
　signs of, 52, 277
　types of, 52, 277
Acceptance of death, 130-131
Accidental poisoning in home, 33
Accidents
　due to equipment, 39
　reporting of, 39
Acetest to test urine for acetone, 169
Acetone in urine, 168
Acquired immunodeficiency syndrome,
　　123-125
　preventing spread of, 29-30
Active-assistive range-of-motion exercises, 259
Activity(ies)
　and bowel elimination, 172
　of daily living, 252
　　observation of, 13
　recreational, 253
　for resident, 276
Adduction, 259
Adjustment, residents', promoting, 43-48
ADL; see Activities of daily living
Admission, 75-77
Admission checklist, 76
Aging
　physical effects of, 45, 46
　psychological and social effects of, 43-45
　social relationships and, 44-45
AIDS; see Acquired immunodeficiency
　　syndrome
AK amputation, 112
AKA, 112
Alcohol and drug use, 6
Alternating pressure mattress to treat
　　decubitus ulcers, 213, 214

Alzheimer's disease, 244-249
　care of resident with, 246, 247-248
　family of resident with, 246, 249
　stages of, 244-246
AM care, 139
Ambulation, 253, 254
Amputation, 112
Anal incontinence, 173
Aneroid sphygmomanometer to measure
　　blood pressure, 72-73
Anger stage of dying, 130
Angina pectoris, 115
Ankle, range-of-motion exercises for, 264
Ankle foot orthoses, 258
Ankle restraint, 37
Antiperspirants, 141
Aphasia, 122
Apical pulse, taking, 68, 69
Apical-radial pulse, taking, 70
Apnea, 70
Appearance of nurse aide, 6
Appetite, observation of, 13
Artery, coronary, disease of, 114-116
Arthritis, 107
Ascending colostomy, 181
Asepsis, 25
　medical, 25-28
Aspergillus, infection or disease caused by,
　　24
Aspiration, prevention of, 148
Asthma, 118
Atherosclerosis, 114-115
Atrophy, muscle, 265
Autoclave, 27, 28
Axillary temperature, taking, 65

B

Back massage, 151, 152
Back rub, 151, 152
Bacteria, 22
　common, infection or disease caused by,
　　24

Bargaining stage of dying, 130
Barrel chest from emphysema, 118, 119
Basic food groups, 188, 189-190
Basic restorative services, 251-272
Bath
　bed, 142-143
　tub, 143
　　shampooing during, 154
Bath blanket, 92
Bath oils, 141
Bathing, 139-143
　general rules for, 142
　grooming, and dressing, 139-158
　observations during, 141-142
Bathroom in resident unit, 88
Bed, 81, 83-85
　Clinitron, to treat decubitus ulcers, 214
　closed, 90, 94
　electric, 83
　Guttmann, to treat decubitus ulcers, 214
　lock on wheel of, 84, 85
　manually operated, 83, 84
　moving resident in, 219-222
　occupied, 90, 91, 94
　open, 90, 91, 94
　positions for, 266-269
　residents in, lifting and moving, 219-227
　shampooing resident in, 154
　side of, moving resident to, 222, 224, 225
　sitting on side of, 227
　turning resident iln, 225-227
Bed bath
　complete, 142-143
　partial, 143
Bed boards, 269
Bed cradle to treat decubitus ulcers, 210, 211
Bed linens, 90, 92-93
Bed rest, 265-271
　complications of, 265
　　preventing, 266
Bedmaking, 89-95
　general rules for, 94
　procedures for, 94-95
Bedpans, 162
Bedside commode, 163
Bedside stand, 85-86
Bedside table, 85-86

Bedsores; see Decubitus ulcers
Bell, tap, 87
Belonging, need for, 236
Below-the-knee amputation, 112
Belt, transfer or gait, 228
　for ambulation, 253, 254
Benign tumors, 126, 127
Between-meal nourishments, 204
BK amputation, 112
Bladder
　observation of, 13
　retraining of, 271
Bland diet, 196
Blanket, bath, 92
Blind resident, locating food on plate for, 204
Blindness, 100-101
Blood pressure, 71-74
　equipment to measure, 72-73
　factors affecting, 71-72
　measuring, 74
Body
　care of, after death, 136
　temperature of; see Temperature
Body mechanics
　general rules for, 217-218
　transfers and, 215-232
　using, 215-218
Body odors, 6
Boiling water for disinfection, 27
Bowel elimination
　factors affecting, 171-172
　normal, 170-171
　observation of, 13
Bowel movement, 171
Bowel retraining, 271
Braces, 258
Bradypnea, 70
Braille, 100
Brain syndrome, chronic, 243-244
Bread and cereal food group, 190
Breath odors, 6
Bronchiectasis, 118
Bronchitis, chronic, 117-118
Brushing
　of hair, 151, 153
　of teeth, 145-147
Burns in home, 32

C

Calcium, 193
Calculi in urinary system, 169-170
Call system in resident unit, 87
Calories in diet, 196, 197
Cancer, 126-128
Candida albicans, infection or disease caused
    by, 24
Canes, 256, 257
Carbohydrates, 190
Cardiovascular system
    changes in, with aging, 46
    problems with, 114-117
Care plan, 18
Caring, 3
Carriers, 23
Carrying, 218
Cast care, 109
Caster, 84, 85
Cataracts, 99
Catheterization, 164
Catheters, 164-166
Centers for Disease Control and infection
    precautions, 28
Centigrade and Fahrenheit equivalents, 58
Centigrade thermometer, 57
Cereal and bread food group, 190
Cerebrovascular accident, 121-122
Chair(s)
    positioning resident in, 266
    in resident unit, 86
    shower, 143, 144
    transferring resident to, 231
Chart, resident's, 17-18
Cheerfulness, 5
Chemical disinfectants, 27
Chemotherapy for cancer, 126
Chest
    barrel, from emphysema, 118, 119
    pain in, 115
Cheyne-Stokes respiration, 70
CHF; *see* Congestive heart failure
Choice, personal, resident's right to, 50,
    274
Chronic brain syndrome, 243-244
Chronic obstructive pulmonary disease,
    117-118
Chyme, 170

Civil laws, 16
"Clean," 29
Clean-catch urine specimen, 167-168
Clean technique, 25
Cleaning of equipment, 26-27
Cleansing enema, 175, 176-177
Clear-liquid diet, 194
Clinical experience, 1
Clinical practicum, 1
Clinical thermometer; *see* Glass thermometer
Clinitest to test urine for sugar, 169
Clinitron bed to treat decubitus ulcers, 214
Closed bed, 90, 94
Closed fracture, 108, 109
Closed reduction of fracture, 109
Closet in resident unit, 88
Code of ethics, 16
Cognitively impaired residents, care of, 243-249
Collection
    of stool specimens, 184
    of urine specimens, 167-170
Colostomy, 180-183
    sites of, 180-181
Colostomy appliance, 182
Coma, diabetic, 120
Comatose resident, mouth care for, 147-149
Combing hair, 151, 153
Comfort
    for dying person, 133-134
    on resident unit, 80-81
Commercial enemas, 175, 177-179
Commodes, 163
Communicable disease, 29, 123-125
Communication, 8-15
    barriers to, 11
    definition of, 8
    with dying resident, 132
    with hearing-impaired person, 102-103
    nonverbal, 11
    with resident, 9-11
    verbal, 9-11
Competency evaluation, nurse aide, 1-2
Complete bed bath, 142-143
Compound fracture, 109
Condom catheter, 166
Conduct, rules of, for nurse aide, 16
Confidentiality, resident's right to, 49-50,
    273-274

Congestive heart failure, 116-117
Conscientiousness, 5
Consent, 17
Consideration, 5
Constipation, 171, 172
Contact lenses, 99
Contagious disease, 29, 123-125
Contamination, 25
Continuous traction, 111
Contracture, 265
Cooperation, 5
COPD; see Chronic obstructive pulmonary
    disease
Coronary artery disease, 114-116
Coronary thrombosis, 115-116
Corrective lenses, 99
Cotton drawsheet, 93
Cough, "smoker's," 117, 118
Courtesy, 5
Creams, 141
Crime, 16
Criminal laws, 16
Culture, 236-237
Curtains in resident unit, 86
Cushion, flotation, to treat decubitus ulcers,
    210, 212
CVA; see Cerebrovascular accident

D

Daily care of resident, 139
Daily living, activities of, 252
    observation of, 13
Dairy product and milk food group, 189
Dangling, 227
Data, objective and subjective, 14
Deafness, 101-103
Death
    acceptance of, 130-131
    approaching, signs of, 135
    attitudes about, 131-132
    care of body after, 136
    signs of, 135
    of spouse, 45
Decubitus ulcers, 207-214
    causes of, 207
    prevention of, 210
    sites of, 207, 208-209
    treatment of, 210-214

Defecation, 171
Delusions, 246, 248
Dementia with Alzheimer's disease, 246,
    248
Denial stage of dying, 130
Dentures
    cleaning, 149-151
    removing, 149
Deodorants, 141
Dependability, 5
Depression about dying, 130
Descending colostomy, 180
Developmental tasks, 237
Diabetes mellitus, 119-120
    testing urine of resident with, 168-170
Diabetic coma, 120
Diabetic diet, 197, 198
Diarrhea, 171, 172
Diastole, 71
Diastolic pressure, 71
Diet(s)
    and bowel elimination, 171-172
    bland, 196
    clear-liquid, 194
    diabetic, 197, 198
    full-liquid, 194
    high-calorie, 196
    high-iron, 195
    high-protein, 197
    high-residue, 195
    liquid, 194
    low-calorie, 197
    low-cholesterol, 197
    low-fat, 197
    low-residue, 195
    sodium-restricted, 193, 198
    soft, 194
    special, 191-198
    therapeutic, common, 194-197
Digestion, problems with, 105-106
"Dirty," 29
Disasters, 41
Discharge, 78
Discomfort, observation of, 12
Disease(s)
    Alzheimer's, 244-249; see also Alzheimer's
        disease
    common, signs and symptoms of, 97-128

Disease(s)—cont'd
  communicable, 29, 123-125
  contagious, 29, 123-125
  coronary artery, 114-116
  lung, 117-119
  Parkinson's, 122-123
  pulmonary, chronic obstructive, 117-118
Disinfection, 25, 27
Disposable equipment, care of, 26
Disposable oral thermometers, 63
Disputes, resident's right to voice, 50, 274
"Do not resuscitate" orders, 135
Dorsiflexion, 259
Double barrel colostomy, 181
Double-voided urine specimen, 168
Drawer space in resident unit, 88
Drawsheet, 92-93
  to move resident to stretcher, 232
Dressing residents, 157
  bathing and grooming and, 139-158
Drinking water, providing, 205
Drug and alcohol use, 6
Dying, stages of, 130-131; *see also* Death
Dying people
  care for, 129-138
  family of, needs of, 134
  physical needs of, 132-134
  psychological, social, and spiritual needs
    of, 132
Dysphagia, 105
Dyspnea, 70
Dysuria, 162

E

Early morning care, 139
Ears, observation of, 12
Eating, factors affecting, 191
Egg crate mattress to treat decubitus ulcers,
  213
Elbow, range-of-motion exercises for, 262
Elbow protectors to treat decubitus ulcers,
  210, 212
Elderly; *see also* Resident(s)
  abuse of, 51-53, 276-278
  sexuality and, 238-240
Electric beds, 83
Electric wire, frayed, 38, 39
Electrical outlet, overloaded, 38, 39

Electronic sphygmomanometer to measure
    blood pressure, 72-73
Electronic talking aid, 9
Electronic thermometers, 61-63
Elimination
  bowel; *see* Bowel elimination
  comfort and safety during, 174
  and dying person, 133
  urinary; *see* Urination
Emergency and safety procedures, 31-42
Empathy, 5
Emphysema, 118
End-of-shift report, 14
Endocrine system, problems with, 119-120
Enema(s), 174-179
  cleansing, 175, 176-177
  commercial, 175, 177-179
  general rules for giving, 176
  oil retention, 175, 179
  saline, 175, 177
  soap solution, 175, 177
  tap water, 175, 177
Enema kits, 175-176
Enema solutions, 175
Enthusiasm, 5
Environment
  of health care facility, 276
  resident's, caring for, 79-96
  safe, 31-32
Equipment
  accidents due to, 39
  cleaning, 26-27
  disposable, care of, 26
  to measure blood pressure, 72-73
  for mouth care, 145
  personal care, in resident unit, 87
  in resident unit, 81-89
Errors, reporting of, 39
Escherichia coli, infection or disease caused
    by, 24
Esteem, need for, 236
Ethics, 16
Evening care, 139
"Exchange lists" for diabetic diet, 198
Exercise(s), 6, 258-264
  range-of-motion, 259-264
Extension, 259
External catheter, 166

External rotation, 259
Eyeglasses, 99
Eyes, observation of, 12

F

Fahrenheit and Centigrade equivalents, 58
Fahrenheit thermometer, 57
Falling resident, supporting, 253, 255
Falls
  in health care facility, preventing, 34-35
  in home, 32
Family
  of dying person, needs of, 134
  of resident, 240
    with Alzheimer's disease, 246, 249
Family groups, resident's right to join, 50,
    274
Fat in diet, 197
Fats, 190-191
Fecal impaction, 173
Fecal incontinence, 173
  bowel retraining for, 271
Feces, 170-171
Feeding resident, 202-204
Feeding techniques, 187-205
Feet, care of, 156
Financial abuse, 52, 277
Fingers, range-of-motion exercises for, 262
Fire
  and oxygen use, 39-40
  prevention of, 40
  procedure for dealing with, 40-41
Fire extinguisher, 41
Fire safety, 39-41
Fish and meat food group, 189
Flatulence, 173-174
Flatus, 173
Flexion, 259
  plantar, footboard to prevent, 270
  radial-ulnar, 259
Flora, normal, 22
Flossing, 147
Flotation pad to treat decubitus ulcers, 210,
    212
Fluid balance, 198-199
Fluids
  and bowel elimination, 172
  and foods, assisting resident with, 202-205

Fluids—cont'd
  "forcing," 199
  restricting, 199
Foam mattress to treat decubitus ulcers, 213
Foley catheter, 164
Folic acid, 192
Food groups, basic, 188, 189-190
Foods and fluids, assisting resident with,
    202-205
Foot, range-of-motion exercises for, 264
Foot restraint, 37
Footboard, 270
Footdrop, footboard to prevent, 270
"Forcing fluids," 199
Forearm, range-of-motion exercises for, 261
Four point cane, 256
Fowler's position, 266
  pressure points in, 209
Fracture(s), 109-111
  closed, 108, 109
  compound, 109
  devices to reduce, 108
  hip, 111
    pinned, 110
  open, 108, 109
  reduction of, 109
  simple, 109
Fracture pan, 162
Frayed electric wire, 38, 39
Fresh-fractional urine specimen, 168
Friction, preventing, when moving resident
    in bed, 219
Fruit and vegetable food group, 189
Full-liquid diet, 194
Fungi, 22
  common, infection or disease caused by,
    24
Furniture in resident unit, 81-89

G

Gait belt, 228
  for ambulation, 253, 254
Gangrene, 112, 113
Gastrointestinal system, 170
  changes in, with aging, 46, 105-106
Germs, 22
Glass thermometer, 57
  cleaning, 58, 60

Glass thermometer—cont'd
  reading, 57, 60
  types of, 57
  using, 58-60, 61
Glasses, 99
Glaucoma, 98
Glucosuria, testing urine to detect, 168-170
Gowns, residents', changing, 157
Graduate to measure fluids, 200
Grievances, resident's right to voice, 50, 274
Grooming, bathing and dressing and, 139-158
Ground, 39
Groups, resident's right to join, 50, 274
Guttman bed to treat decubitus ulcers, 214

H

Hair
  brushing and combing, 151, 153
  care of, 151, 153-154
  shampooing, 153-154
Hallucinations, 246, 248
Hand rails, 34
Hand restraint, 37
Handwashing, 25-27
Head
  injuries of, 104
  and shoulders of resident, raising, 219, 220
Health
  mental, 236
    needs involving, 233-241
  personal, of nurse aid, 6
Health care facility
  environment of, 276
  falls in, preventing, 34-35
  safety in, 33-35
Hearing
  during dying process, 132-133
  problems with, 101-103
Hearing aids, 103, 104
Hearing-impaired person, communicating
    with, 102-103
Heart attack, 115-116
Heart failure, congestive, 116-117
Heel protectors to treat decubitus ulcers,
    210, 212
Height, measurement of, on admission, 75
Hemiplegia, 122
Hepatitis, 125

Hepatitis A, 125
  infection or disease caused by, 24
Hepatitis B, 125
  infection or disease caused by, 24
Herpes simplex I, infection or disease
    caused by, 24
High-calorie diet, 196
High-iron diet, 195
High-protein diet, 197
High-residue diet, 195
Hip
  fracture of, 111
    pinning, 110, 111
  range-of-motion exercises for, 263
HIV, infection or disease caused by, 24
Home, safety in, 32-33
Honesty, 5
Hospice care, 134-135
Host, 22
  susceptibility of, 23
HS care, 139
Hygiene
  of nurse aide, 6
  oral, 145-151
  personal, 139-156
Hyperextension, 259
Hypertension, 71, 114
Hyperventilation, 70
Hypotension, 71-72
Hypoventilation, 70

I

Identification of resident, 33-34
Identification bracelets for resident, 33
Ileostomy, 183-184
Ileostomy appliance, 184
Illness
  psychological and social effects of, 237
  terminal, 130
Immobility, complications of, 265
Immunodeficiency syndrome, acquired,
    123-125
Impaction, fecal, 173
Incident reports, 39
Incontinence
  fecal, 173
  retraining for, 271
  urinary, 166-167

Independence, residents', promoting, 43-48
Indwelling catheter, 164
Infarction, myocardial, 115-116
Infection, 22-24
    chain of, 23
    process of, 23
Infection control, 21-30
Infection precautions, 28-30
Infectious diseases, 123-125
Infectious hepatitis, 125
Informed consent, 17
Infusions, IV, changing gown of resident
        with, 157
Insulin shock, 120
Intake and output
    measuring, 200-202
    records of, 199-202
Integumentary changes with aging, 47
Intermittent traction, 111
Internal rotation, 259
Invasion of privacy, 17
Involuntary seclusion, 52, 277
I&O; see Intake and output
Iodine, 193
Iron, 193
    increasing, in diet, 195
Isolation techniques, 28
IV infusions, changing gown of resident
        with, 157

J
Jacket restraint, 36, 37
Jewelry for nurse aide, 6
Joints, problems with, 106-107

K
Kardex, nursing care plan in, 18-19
Keto-Diastix to test urine for sugar and
        acetone, 169
Ketone bodies in urine, 168
Ketones in urine, 168
Knee, range-of-motion exercises for, 263

L
Language, sign, 10
Lateral position, 267, 268
    pressure points in, 208
Law, 16

Leg brace, 258
Leg prosthesis, 113
Legal considerations, 16-17
Lenses, corrective, 99
Liability, 17
Life, quality of, of resident, 276
Lift sheet, moving resident up in bed using,
        222, 223
Lifting, 217
    and moving residents in bed, 219-227
Lifts, mechanical, 231-232
Lighting of resident unit, 81
Limb, loss of, 112-114
Linens, bed, 90, 92-93
Liquid diet, 194
Listening, 11
Living, daily, activities of, 252
    observation of, 13
Living wills, 135
Lock on bed wheel, 84, 85
Logrolling, 227
Lotions, 141
Love, need for, 236
Low-calorie diet, 197
Low-cholesterol diet, 197
Low-fat diet, 197
Low-residue diet, 195
Lower leg prosthesis, 113
Lung diseases, 117-119

M
Malignant tumors, 126, 127
Malpractice, 17
Manometer to measure blood pressure, 72
Manually operated bed, 83, 84
Massage, back, 151, 152
Mattresses to treat decubitus ulcers, 213-214
Meal trays, serving, 202, 203
Meats and fish food group, 189
Mechanical lifts, 231-232
Medical asepsis, 25-28
Medications and bowel elimination, 172
Mental abuse, 52, 277
    freedom from, resident's right to, 51
Mental health, 236
    and social service needs, 233-241
Mercury sphygmomanometer to measure
        blood pressure, 72-73

Metastasis of cancer, 126
MI; *see* Myocardial infarction
Microbes, 21
Microorganisms, 21-22
Micturation; *see* Urination
Milk and dairy products food group, 189
Minerals, 191
    functions and sources of, 193
Mistreatment, freedom from, resident's
        right to, 51, 275
Mitt restraint, 37
Morning care, 139
Mouth
    care of, 145-151
        for dying person, 133
        for unconscious or comatose resident,
            147-149
    observation of, 12
Movement, observation of, 12
Moving resident
    in bed, 219-222
        lifting resident and, 219-227
    to side of bed, 222, 224, 225
    to stretcher, 232
MS; *see* Multiple sclerosis
Multiple sclerosis, 123
Muscle, atrophy of, 265
Musculoskeletal system, changes in, with
        aging, 46, 106-114
Myocardial infarction, 115-116

N
Nails, care of, 156
Neck, range-of-motion exercises for, 261
Needs, 234-236
    esteem, 236
    love and belonging, 236
    Maslow's hierarchy of, 235
    physiological, 234-235
    safety and security, 235-236
    self-actualization, 236
Neglect, freedom from, resident's right to,
        51, 275
Negligence, 16, 17
Neisseria gonorrheae, infection or disease
        caused by, 24
Nervous system
    changes in, with aging, 47

Nervous system—cont'd
    disorders of, 121-123
Niacin, 192
"No code" orders, 135
Noise in resident unit, 80-81
Nonpathogens, 21
Nonverbal communication, 11
Normal flora, 22
Nose
    care of, for dying person, 133
    observation of, 12
Nourishment, between-meal, 204
NPO, 199
Nurse aide
    competency evaluation for, 1-2
    conduct of, 16
    ethical and legal considerations for, 15-17
    functions and responsibilities of, 6-8
    personal health, hygiene, and appearance
        of, 6
    practical training for, 1
    qualities and characteristics of, 3-5
    registry for, 2
    training program for, 1-2
Nursing care plan, 18
Nursing facilities, 45, 48
Nursing homes, 45, 48
Nutrients, 190-191
Nutrition, 6, 189-190
    factors affecting, 191

O
Objective data, 14
OBRA; *see* Omnibus Budget Reconciliation
        Act
Observations, 14
    during bathing, 141-142
    reporting and recording, 11-15
    of resident, 12-13
Occlusion, coronary, 115-116
Occupied bed, 90, 91, 94
Odors
    body and breath, 6
    in resident unit, 80
Oil retention enema, 175, 179
Oils, bath, 141
Omnibus Budget Reconciliation Act, 1
    on resident rights, 15

Open bed, 90, 91, 94
Open fracture, 108, 109
Open reduction of fracture, 109
Opposition, thumb, 259
Oral hygiene, 145-151
Oral temperatures, taking, 63
Oral thermometers, disposable, 63
Orthoses, ankle foot, 258
Orthotic devices, care of, 272
Osteoarthritis, 107
Osteoporosis, 112
  causing fractures, 109
Ostomy, resident with, 179-184
Outlet, electrical, overloaded, 38, 39
Output, intake and
  measuring, 200-202
  records of, 199-202
Overbed table, 85
Overloaded electrical outlet, 38, 39
Oxygen, fire and use of, 39-40

P
Pain
  chest, 115
  observation of, 12
  phantom limb, 114
Paralysis, 104-105
Paraplegia, 105
Parkinson's disease, 122-123
Partial bath, 143
Passive range-of-motion exercises, 259
Pathogens, 21
  transmission of, 23
Pericare, 144-145
Perineal care, 144-145
Peristalsis, 170-171
Personal care equipment in resident unit, 87
Personal choice, resident's right to, 50, 274
Personal health of nurse aide, 6
Personal hygiene, 139-156
Personal possessions, resident's right to care
  and security of, 50-51, 275
Phantom limb pain, 114
Phosphorus, 193
Physical abuse, 52, 277
  freedom from, resident's right to, 51
Physiological needs, 234-235
Pinning, hip, 110, 111

Plantar flexion, footboard to prevent, 270
Plasmodium falciparum, infection or disease
  caused by, 24
Plastic covers for thermometers, 59, 60
Plastic drawsheet, 92
Plug, three pronged, 38, 39
Pneumonia, 118-119
Poisoning, accidental, in home, 33
Portal of entry and exit for pathogens, 23
Positioning
  aids for, 269-271
  of dying person, 133-134
  of resident in chair, 266
Positions, bed, 266-269
Possessions, personal, resident's right to
  care and security of, 50-51, 275
Postmortem care, 136
Potassium, 193
Powders, 141
Practical training for nurse aide, 1
Pressure
  blood, 71-74; *see also* Blood pressure
  steam under, for disinfection, 28
Pressure points and decubitus ulcers,
  208-209
Pressure sores; *see* Decubitus ulcers
Privacy
  and bowel elimination, 171
  invasion of, 17
  resident's right to, 49-50, 273-274
Pronation, 259
Prone position, 267, 268
  pressure points in, 208
Prosthesis, 112-114
Prosthetic devices, care of, 272
Protective devices, 35-37, 39
Protein, 190
  in diet, 196, 197
Protozoa, 22
  common, infection or disease caused by,
  24
Pulmonary disease, chronic obstructive,
  117-118
Pulse, 66
  apical, taking, 68, 69
  apical-radial, taking, 70
  measuring, 66-70
  radial, taking, 68, 69

Pulse—cont'd
  rhythm and force of, 66
  sites for taking, 66, 68-70
Pulse deficit, 70
Pulse rate, 66

Q

Quad cane, 256
Quadriplegia, 105
Quality of life of resident, 276

R

Radial-apical pulse, taking, 70
Radial pulse, taking, 68, 69
Radial-ulnar flexion, 259
"Radiation sickness," 126
Radiation therapy for cancer, 126
Radiotherapy for cancer, 126
Raising head and shoulders of resident,
    219, 220
Range-of-motion exercises, 259-264
Reality orientation, 244
Reality orientation board, 244
Record(s)
  intake and output, 199-202
  resident's, 17-18
Recording, 11, 14-15
  of height and weight on admission,
    76
  of restraint use, 37
Recreational activities, 253
Rectal temperature, taking, 64, 65
Reduction of fracture, 109
Registry, nurse aide, 2
Rehabilitation, 271-272
Reincarnation, 131
Religion, 237
  and atitudes about death, 131
Report(s)
  end-of-shift, 14
  incident, 39
Reporting, 11, 14
  of accidents and errors, 39
  on restraint use, 37
  on vital signs, 55-56
Reproductive system, changes in, with
    aging, 47, 106
Reservoir, 22, 23

Resident(s), 48
  activities for, 276
  adjustment, independence, and rights of,
    promoting, 43-48
  with Alzheimer's disease, care of, 246,
    247-248
  in bed, lifting and moving, 219-227
  cognitively impaired, care of,
    243-249
  communicating with, 9-11
  daily care of, 139
  dressing and undressing, 157
  dying, care for, 129-138
  environment of, caring for, 79-96
  falling, supporting, 253, 255
  family and visitors of, 240
  feeding, 202-204
  identifying, 33-34
  moving
    in bed, 219-222
    to side of bed, 222, 224, 225
    to stretcher, 232
  observations of, 12-13
  rights of, 273-278
    promoting, 15
    respecting, 49-53
  sexually aggressive, 239-240
  transferring of, 227-232
    to chair or wheelchair, 231
  turning, in bed, 225-227
  unconscious or comatose, mouth care for,
    147-149
Resident groups, resident's right to join, 50,
    274
Resident unit, 79, 82
  comfort on, 80-81
  of dying person, 134
  furniture and equipment in, 81-89
  general rules for, 89
Resident's record, 17-18
Respectfulness, 5
Respirations, 70-71
  observation of, 13
Respiratory system
  changes in, with aging, 46
  problems with, 117-119
Responsibility, 6
Responsiveness, observation of, 12

Rest
  bed; *see* Bed rest
  sleep and, 6
Restorative services, basic, 251-272
Restraints, 35-37, 39
  freedom from, resident's right to, 51,
    275-276
Retention catheter, 164
Retirement, 44
Reverse Trendelenburg's position, 267
Rheumatoid arthritis, 107
Riboflavin, 192
Rickettsia rickettsii, infection or disease
  caused by, 24
Rickettsiae, 22
  common, infection or disease caused by,
    24
Rights, residents', 273-278
  promoting, 15, 43-48
  respecting, 49-53
Rigor mortis, 136
ROM; *see* Range-of-motion exercises
Rotation, 259
  external, 259
  internal, 259
Routine urine specimens, 167
Rubber drawsheet, 92

S
Safe environment, 31-32
Safety
  and emergency procedures, 31-42
  during elimination, 174
  fire, 39-41
  in health care facility, 33-35
  in home, 32-33
Safety belt, 39
Safety needs, 235-236
Saline enema, 175, 177
Sclerosis, multiple, 123
Screens in resident unit, 86
Seclusion, involuntary, 52, 277
Security needs, 235-236
Self-actualization, need for, 236
Self-awareness, 5
Self-help devices, 252
Semi-Fowler's position, 267
Serum hepatitis, 125

Sexual abuse, 52, 277
  freedom from, resident's right to, 51
Sexuality and elderly, 238-240
Sexually aggressive resident, 239-240
Shampooing, 153-154
Shaving, 155
Sheepskin to treat decubitus ulcers, 210,
  211
Sheet, turning (lift), moving resident up in
  bed using, 222, 223
Shock, insulin, 120
Shoulder(s)
  and head of resident, raising, 219, 220
  range-of-motion exercises for, 261
Shower, 143
  shampooing during, 154
Shower chair, 143, 144
"Sickness, radiation," 126
Side-lying position, 267, 268
Side rails, 34
Sigmoid colostomy, 180
Sign language, 10
Signs, 14
Simple fracture, 109
Sim's position, 268, 269
  for giving enema, 177
Single tipped cane, 256
Sink, shampooing at, 154
Sitting on side of bed, 227
Sitting position, pressure points in, 209
Skin
  care of, 207-214
    for dying person, 133
  observation of, 12
Skin-care products, 141
Sleep and rest, 6
"Smoker's cough," 117, 118
Smoking, 6
Snacks, 204
Soap solution enema, 175, 177
Soaps, 141
Social relationships of elderly, 44-45
Social service and mental health needs,
  233-241
Sodium, 193
Sodium-restricted diet, 193, 198
Soft diet, 194
Solutions, enema, 175

Sores, pressure; *see* Decubitus ulcers
Special diets, 191-198
Specimens
   stool, collecting, 184
   urine, collecting and testing, 167-170
Speech during dying process, 132-133
Speech impairments, 103
Sphygmomanometer to measure blood
     pressure, 72
Spinal cord injuries, 104-105
Spores, 27
Spouse, death of, 45
Staphylococcus aureus, infection or disease
     caused by, 24
Steam under pressure for disinfection, 28
Sterile, 25
Sterilization, 25, 27-28
Stethoscope, 66, 67
   to measure blood pressure, 72
   using, 66
Stoma, 179
Stomatitis, 126
Stones in urinary system, 169-170
Stool, 171
Stool specimens, collecting, 184
Straining of urine, 169-170
Streptococcus, infection or disease caused by,
   24
Stretcher
   moving resident to, 232
   shampooing resident on, 154
Stroke, 121-122
Stump conditioning, 112, 114
Subjective data, 14
Suffocation, 33
Sundowning, 246, 247-248
Supination, 259
Supine position, 267
   pressure points in, 208
Suppository, 271
Susceptibility of host, 23
Swallowing, difficulty in, 105
Symptoms, 14
Syndrome
   acquired immunodeficiency, 123-125
   brain, chronic, 243-244
Systole, 71
Systolic pressure, 71

T
Table
   bedside, 85-86
   overbed, 85
Tachypnea, 70
Talking aid, electronic, 9
Tap bell, 87
Tap water enema, 175, 177
Teeth
   brushing, 145-147
   flossing, 147
"Temp board," 56
Temperature
   axillary, taking, 65
   body
      measuring, 56-65
      normal, 56
   oral, taking, 63
   rectal, taking, 64, 65
   of resident unit, 80
Terminal illness, 130
Testape to test urine for sugar, 169
Testing of urine specimens, 167-170
Texas catheter, 166
Therapeutic diets, common, 194-197
Thermometer, 56
   electronic, 61-63
   glass; *see* Glass thermometer
   oral, disposable, 63
   plastic cover for, 59, 60
Thiamin, 192
Three pronged plug, 38, 39
Thrombosis, coronary, 115-116
Thumb
   opposition of, 259
   range-of-motion exercises for, 263
Toes, range-of-motion exercises for,
   264
Toileting, 159-185
Toothette, 145
"TPR book," 56
Traction, 111
Traction set-up, 110
   with trapeze, 259
Training, practical, for nurse aide, 1
Training program, nurse aide, 1-2
Transfer belt, 228
   for ambulation, 253, 254

Transferring of residents, 227-232
  to chair or wheelchair, 231
Transfers and body mechanics, 215-232
Transmission of pathogen, 23
Transverse colostomy, 181
Trapeze, 258, 259
Trendelenburg's position, 267
Tri-pod cane, 256
Trochanter rolls, 270, 271
Trustworthiness, 5
Tub bath, 143
  shampooing during, 154
Tumor, 126, 127
Tunnel vision, 98
Turning residents in bed, 225-227
Turning sheet, moving resident up in bed
    using, 222, 223
24-hour urine specimen, 168

U

Ulcers, decubitus, 207-214; *see also*
    Decubitus ulcers
Undressing residents, 157
  mouth care for, 147-149
Universal precautions, 29-30
Urinal, 163
Urinary incontinence, 166-167
  bladder retraining for, 271
Urinary system, 159, 160
  changes in, with aging, 46, 121
Urination
  frequency of, 161
  normal, 159-161
    maintaining, 161-163
Urine, straining, 169-170
Urine specimens
  clean-catch, 167-168
  collecting and testing, 167-170
  double-voided or fresh-fractional, 168

Urine specimens—cont'd
  routine, 167
  24-hour, 168

V

Vegetable and fruit food group, 189
Ventilation of resident unit, 80
Verbal abuse, 52, 277
  freedom from, resident's right to, 51
Verbal communication, 9-11
Viruses, 22
  common, infection or disease caused by,
    24
Vision
  during dying process, 132-133
  problems with, 98-101
Visitors, 240
Vital signs, 55-74
  measuring and reporting, 55-56
Vitamins, 191
  functions and sources of, 192
Voiding; *see* Urination

W

Waist restraint, 39
Walkers, 257-258
Walking aids, 257-264
Wandering, 245-246, 247
Water
  drinking, providing, 205
  normal requirements for, 199
Water balance, 198-199
Water beds to treat decubitus ulcers, 213
Weight, measurement of, on admission, 75,
    77
Wheelchair, transferring resident to, 231
Wills, living, 135
Wrist, range-of-motion exercises for, 262
Wrist restraint, 37